The Athlete's Guide to

MAKING
WEIGHT

The Athlete's Guide to

MAKING WEIGHT

Michele A. Macedonio, MS, RD
Marie Dunford, PhD, RD

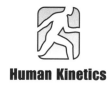

Human Kinetics

Library of Congress Cataloging-in-Publication Data

Macedonio, Michele A.
  The athlete's guide to making weight / Michele A. Macedonio, Marie Dunford.
      p. cm.
  Includes bibliographical references and index.
  ISBN-13: 978-0-7360-7586-2 (soft cover)
  ISBN-10: 0-7360-7586-0 (soft cover)
  1. Sports--Physiological aspects. 2. Athletes--Nutrition. 3. Body weight--Regulation. 4. Sports medicine.
I. Dunford, Marie. II. Title.
  RC1235.M26 2009
  613.2'024796--dc22
                                          2008052163

ISBN-10: 0-7360-7586-0 (print)   ISBN-10: 0-7360-8524-6 (Adobe PDF)
ISBN-13: 978-0-7360-7586-2 (print)   ISBN-13: 978-0-7360-8524-3 (Adobe PDF)

This publication is written and published to provide accurate and authoritative information relevant to the subject matter presented. It is published and sold with the understanding that the author and publisher are not engaged in rendering legal, medical, or other professional services by reason of their authorship or publication of this work. If medical or other expert assistance is required, the services of a competent professional person should be sought.

The Web addresses cited in this text were current as of October 2008, unless otherwise noted.

Developmental Editor: Heather Healy; **Assistant Editor:** Carla Zych; **Copyeditor:** Robert Replinger; **Proofreader:** Kathy Bennett; **Indexer:** Nan N. Badgett; **Permission Manager:** Martha Gullo; **Graphic Designer:** Robert Reuther; **Graphic Artist:** Kim McFarland; **Cover Designer:** Keith Blomberg; **Photographer (cover):** © Human Kinetics; **Photographer (interior):** © Human Kinetics unless otherwise indicated; **Photo Asset Manager:** Laura Fitch; **Photo Production Manager:** Jason Allen; **Art Manager:** Kelly Hendren; **Associate Art Manager:** Alan L. Wilborn; **Illustrator:** Figure 3.1 by Mic Greenberg; all others by Gary Hunt; **Printer:** United Graphics

Human Kinetics books are available at special discounts for bulk purchase. Special editions or book excerpts can also be created to specification. For details, contact the Special Sales Manager at Human Kinetics.

Printed in the United States of America   10 9 8 7 6 5 4 3 2 1

Human Kinetics
Web site: www.HumanKinetics.com

United States: Human Kinetics
P.O. Box 5076
Champaign, IL 61825-5076
800-747-4457
e-mail: humank@hkusa.com

Canada: Human Kinetics
475 Devonshire Road Unit 100
Windsor, ON N8Y 2L5
800-465-7301 (in Canada only)
e-mail: info@hkcanada.com

Europe: Human Kinetics
107 Bradford Road
Stanningley
Leeds LS28 6AT, United Kingdom
+44 (0) 113 255 5665
e-mail: hk@hkeurope.com

Australia: Human Kinetics
57A Price Avenue
Lower Mitcham, South Australia 5062
08 8372 0999
e-mail: info@hkaustralia.com

New Zealand: Human Kinetics
Division of Sports Distributors NZ Ltd.
P.O. Box 300 226 Albany
North Shore City
Auckland
0064 9 448 1207
e-mail: info@humankinetics.co.nz

*To my parents, Annette and Carmine, who believed I could,
and to my husband, Matt, who knew I would.*

—MM

To my husband, Greg, from whom all good things flow.

—MD

Contents

Preface

Andre Agassi, a professional tennis player by age 16, was a rebel with shoulder-length hair, a cheeseburger-heavy diet, and camera ads that proclaimed, "Image is everything." He had many successes early in his career, but after 10 years the former number 1 player was ranked 141st and playing on the satellite tour. His options were to quit or improve. He shaved his head, changed his image, rededicated himself to a rigorous training and conditioning program, and revamped his diet. In doing so, he changed his weight and body composition. Agassi discovered a balance between the demands of the sport, his skills and style of play, and the physical and nutritional preparation essential to achieving long-term success. The rest is history.

If you are serious about your sport and aspire to peak performance, you need to be aware of how body weight and composition affect performance. Whether you are a basketball player looking to increase size and power for an improved inside game or a wrestler debating the advantages of dropping to a lower weight class, *The Athlete's Guide to Making Weight* provides the information that you need to determine where you are, where you need to be, and how you are going to get there.

This book is a guide to help you answer questions about weight and performance. Should I lose weight? Should I gain weight? If so, how? What are the advantages of adding muscle or losing fat? How can I do so without jeopardizing my performance? How does water weight factor in, and what role do supplements play in the overall process? Combining the latest research and real-life examples, along with sample meal plans and sport-specific programming, this book provides the answers to these sorts of questions and puts you on the road to successful weight loss or gain.

The Athlete's Guide to Making Weight leads the dedicated athlete through a logical and thoughtful process of change. The book is designed to help you determine the best weight and body composition for your sport and position. The book begins with an explanation of the four steps needed to achieve optimal performance weight so that you can briefly see the overall process that will help you meet your goals. In part I you learn about assessments and goal setting. Assessment is essential, so three chapters are devoted to it. Chapter 1 helps you assess the relative need for strength, power, speed, and endurance in different sports and how weight and body composition affect these characteristics. To set realistic goals and objectives to improve your performance, you need to complete a comprehensive assessment of your sport and yourself. Chapter 2 presents priorities for your sport and your specific position, and chapter 3 explains the personal assessments that will help you establish a baseline for your body.

Part II begins with a primer on nutrition (chapter 4) because proper nutrition is a crucial support to training. In the quest to change weight and body composition, many people focus too much on the amount of calories found in food. Caloric intake is important, but you cannot afford to overlook the nutrients that foods provide. Chapter 5 explains how caloric intake and nutrients work together to fuel the body. Chapters 6, 7, and 8 provide information about how to build muscle, lose fat, and maintain proper hydration. Misinformation about these processes can lead to unrealistic or inappropriate goals and action plans that can be detrimental to your training, performance, and health. Chapter 9 evaluates many of the dietary supplements that are advertised to help athletes build muscle and lose body fat.

Part III contains specific action plans for achieving your goals. You will find meal plans to help you build muscle (chapter 10), lose fat (chapter 11), or build muscle and lose fat at the same time (chapter 12). These nutritionally sound meal plans include the proper amounts and proportions of calories, carbohydrate, protein, and fat. In chapter 13 you will learn how to personalize your meal plan and create daily meal patterns (meals and snacks) that support your training and conditioning program.

Changing weight and body composition is a step-by-step process, so we recommend that you read the introduction and then begin with the assessments in part I. You may be tempted to start with part III, but without a detailed assessment of where you are now and what you need to do to improve your performance in your sport and at your position, you could easily choose the wrong calorie level and meal plan. Begin at the beginning, and you will see the results that you desire in the end.

Acknowledgments

Life takes us down many paths, and along the way we are blessed to encounter people who help to shape us. My parents, Annette and Carmine Macedonio, always believed in me and encouraged me to push my limits. They planted the seeds for this book and for all my accomplishments, and I only wish they could have enjoyed the fruit.

I could not have had a more perfect co-author than Marie Dunford, who not only helped me realize a dream but also made the process enjoyable and exciting. This project strengthened our friendship and increased my admiration for Marie.

I'm grateful to Jason Muzinic at Human Kinetics for presenting the challenge and for having faith in us, trusting us to reach the goal line.

Many thanks to my friends Janet Thomas and Lisa Schackmann for their expert eyes and insightful suggestions early in the writing process, which helped us speak more clearly to our readers.

Thanks, too, to my wonderful clients, especially Rudi Johnson, Landon Johnson, Erin Mikula, Evan Schwinfest, Jill Glassmeyer, Colin Cotton, and Justin Haire, who have faithfully followed my counsel, given me inspiration, and proven that this method works.

Special thanks to Heather Healy and the entire HK editorial and production team for their support, encouragement, expertise, and creativity in fine-tuning this work.

To my family—my husband, Matt Sokany; my children, Katherine and Morgan; and my Aunt Mickey—thanks for being my biggest fans. And to all who have helped me reach this place—thank you!

—Michele Macedonio

Jason Muzinic has long held a vision for a book about athletes and weight, and I thank him for trusting me to be a part of it.

Michele Macedonio is a phenomenal co-author. Although we have known each other for years, only in writing this book did we discover that we are twin daughters of different mothers.

Thanks to Mike Newell for critiquing the chapters and dropping them off on his early morning dog walks.

This book would not have been possible without Heather Healy and the other members of the editorial and production team, who expertly transformed the manuscript to its final form.

To all those named and unnamed, thank you for your help and encouragement.

—Marie Dunford

Introduction

Four Steps to Achieving Optimal Performance Weight

Like many people, athletes often look to quick fixes, crash diets, or shortcuts to achieve weight loss or weight gain. You may have already tried some of those methods and found that they did not work or that they hindered your performance. Athletes who want to gain or lose weight and change body composition to improve performance need to understand that achieving that end is a process. A process is a series of well-thought-out actions directed toward specific goals. Athletes work on at least three goals simultaneously: a performance-based goal, a weight and body-composition goal, and a health-based goal. Each step of the process builds on a previous step until the goals are achieved. Although each athlete needs a personalized plan to meet individualized goals, the process is the same.

To help you understand the process, we have created a four-step approach that will help you achieve the performance improvements you want. Step 1 is *assessment*, a necessary precondition to understanding your situation. After you have assessment information, you can proceed to *goal setting* (step 2). Realistic performance, weight, and health goals and objectives are the basis for creating an *action plan*, which is step 3. Many athletes are unsuccessful in their attempts at weight loss or gain because they jump into an action plan that is not based on realistic goals that suit their unique needs. Step 4 is *evaluation and reassessment*, an important step because strategies often need to be adjusted and because goals, objectives, and priorities change.

Step 1: Assessment

Assessment focuses on two specific areas: an assessment of your sport and a personal assessment. You must have a clear understanding of your sport and position and be aware of the height, weight, body build, and body composition of successful athletes in your sport. Personal assessments that evaluate your physical characteristics are critical because they serve as baseline measurements. You need to measure your height, weight, body build, girth, and body composition as well as your calorie intake and expenditure.

By comparing your physical characteristics with those of successful athletes in your sport, specifically with those who play your position, you can determine whether you need to change your body weight or body composition. Most athletes find that they need to make some changes. Because you cannot make these changes without altering your current caloric intake (that is, your diet) or your current caloric expenditure (your exercise), the recording of these data provides valuable baseline information. You will have to devote some time to obtain the measurements needed. This time is well spent because assessment gives you the baseline information that you need to set realistic goals and objectives.

Step 2: Goal Setting

When an athlete says, "I want to lose weight" or "I want to gain muscle mass," he or she is setting a goal. Such broad goals keep you focused on the prize of improving your performance. You may want to gain weight as muscle so that you are bigger and stronger and can overpower an opponent, you may want to lose excess body fat to increase your speed, or you may want to maximize muscle and minimize fat to successfully compete in a lower weight class. Whatever your goal, to accomplish it, you need to take many small steps. These small steps, known as objectives, need to be specific. For example, if your goal is to gain 20 pounds (9 kilograms) of muscle mass, then one objective should be the amount of lean mass that you hope to gain at one-month intervals. Gaining 20 pounds (9 kilograms) of muscle mass may take a year, so objectives are minigoals that can help you stay on track. Athletes usually have several major goals and numerous objectives. After you set goals and objectives, you can institute an action plan.

Step 3: Action Plan

To make a change, you should understand the current situation and have a specific plan to meet your goals. Basic nutrition knowledge is critical because you need proper nutrition for optimal training, performance, and good health. Knowing how muscle is gained and how body fat is lost is prerequisite information for your action plan because you do not want to make changes that impede progress toward your goals or interfere with your training and performance. Changing weight or body composition requires you to modify your diet, and dietary intake is a primary focus of any action plan. Your plan should include the specific amounts of calories, carbohydrate, protein, and fat that you need to consume daily.

Step 4: Evaluation and Reassessment

Evaluation and reassessment are necessary to determine whether you are meeting your goals and objectives and whether your action plan is working. Remember, you will set goals that relate to performance, weight and body composition, and health, and you need to evaluate your progress to see if the results are those you intended. You will have to repeat many of the personal assessments originally conducted because you will need comparative measurements to judge whether you are achieving your goals and objectives. This step provides valuable feedback and can lead to adjustments in your goals and objectives and modifications to the strategies needed to meet them. Changes in weight and body composition cannot be precisely predicted. Even a well-developed action plan will likely need adjustment along the way.

The illustration of the four steps to achieving optimal performance weight in figure 1 on page 4 gives you an overview of the process and shows how each step builds on the previous ones. As you can see, each chapter in the book gives specific information about one or more of the steps. Personalizing this process will help you determine and achieve your optimal performance weight. Here's to your success!

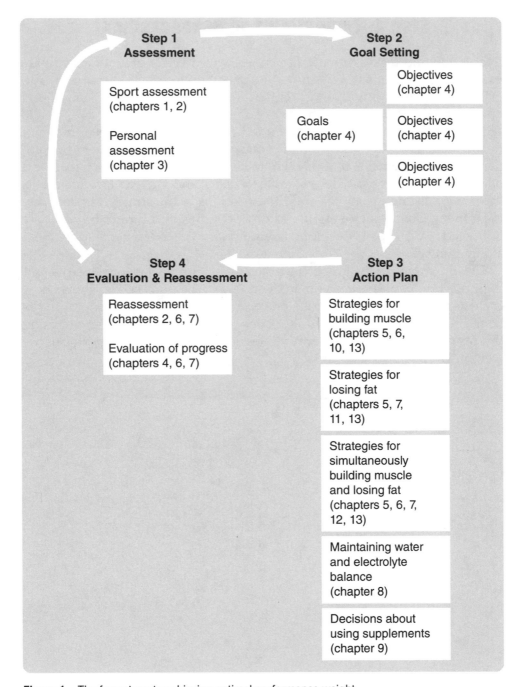

Figure 1   The four steps to achieving optimal performance weight.

PART I

Optimal Weight,
Optimal Performance

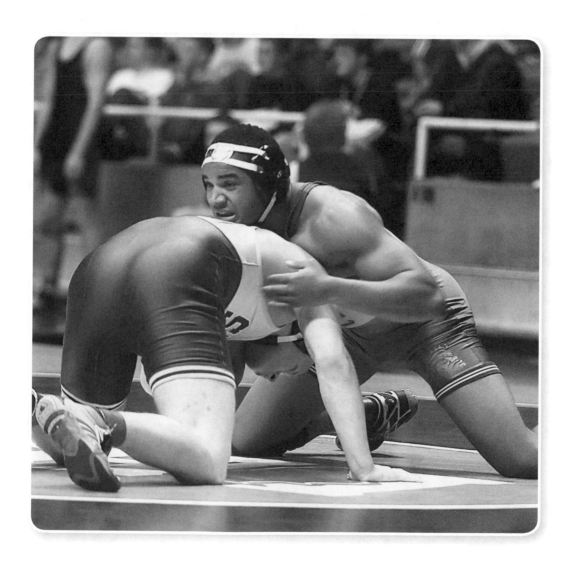

Tipping the Scales in Your Favor

What is your optimal performance weight? The answer largely depends on your sport and the position that you play. The right weight and body composition reflect the physiological demands of your sport and position and your genetic makeup. Understanding the physical characteristics of successful athletes in your sport will help you identify your best weight and body composition. Although individual differences must always be accommodated, certain body characteristics are advantageous in particular sports.

Take a moment to think about the physical characteristics of outstanding athletes in your sport. How tall are they? How much do they typically weigh? Do they have a large amount of muscle mass? Do they have a relatively low percentage of body fat? Assessing your sport will give you a basis for comparing your body to successful athletes in your sport. Consider whether you would perform better if you had more muscle. At what level would muscle mass become excessive and thus be detrimental to performance? Conversely, would your performance improve if you had less body fat, and if so, how much? Keep in mind that losing too much fat undermines performance. By asking yourself these questions you will begin to understand whether you need to gain or lose weight and whether you need more lean mass or less body fat to perform at your peak.

Four factors that you must consider when assessing your sport are height, weight, body build, and body composition. These physical parameters relate to size, and size is related to success in most sports. In many sports, becoming bigger by adding more weight, especially as muscle, can be advantageous. Some sports, however, favor lightweight bodies, so athletes competing in those activities may benefit by losing weight or maintaining a low percentage of body fat. The relative need for power and endurance strongly influences optimal performance weight, and athletes must identify the appropriate balance between the amount of muscle needed to produce power and the additional weight that results from added muscle mass.

Strength, Power, Speed, and Endurance

Some terms frequently used in athletics include *strength*, *power*, *speed*, and *endurance*. In everyday language these terms have a variety of meanings, but exercise physiologists use precise definitions. This book uses the following definitions in application to athletics:

Strength. The maximal force that muscle can generate

Power. The explosive aspect of strength; a function of both strength and speed

Speed. The rate of movement; distance divided by time

Endurance. The ability to resist fatigue; more often refers to cardiovascular endurance (for example, endurance athletes) but can also refer to muscle endurance

Sport-specific physical demands dictate, to a degree, the amount of muscle mass or body fat that is well matched to that sport.

Size

Size refers to both height and weight. Size is a factor in many sports, especially certain positions in contact sports. Larger physical size can result in greater strength, longer stride length, and the ability to cover more area and see over other players. In basketball, height and weight are an advantage for a center who uses size to score and defend near the basket. For a soccer goalie, height offers an advantage in protecting a greater area of the goal, but extra weight could slow response time. Conversely, smaller players in contact sports may be overpowered or physically harmed. In sports such as wrestling or boxing, weight categories exist because larger athletes would have an overwhelming advantage over smaller athletes.

In football, linemen who are both "big" and strong have an advantage. Offensive linemen use their size and strength to move the defensive line back, protect the quarterback, and create holes for the running back. A defensive lineman can overpower an offensive lineman who lacks size. Offensive linemen who play in the National Football League (NFL) are large. Most weigh over 300 pounds (136 kilograms) so that they can match up with their defensive counterparts. Much of this weight is muscle, bone, and fluid, but some of it is fat.

Achieving Proper Body Composition

Physical size is only one aspect of optimal weight; achieving proper body composition is another. In contact sports, a large athlete who lacks sufficient muscle mass will not have the strength needed to perform well. Excessive body fat can negatively affect speed and fitness, but too little body fat can create a size disadvantage. Weight and body composition are both factors in athletic success.

For example, offensive and defensive linemen typically have a higher percentage of body fat than other players on the football team because greater body weight and size are important factors in their performance and their positions do not require them to run across a large portion of the field. Extra body fat can be advantageous if it contributes to size without diminishing strength, speed, or flexibility. But excess body fat can interfere with mobility, create orthopedic problems, and contribute to sleep apnea (a temporary stoppage of breathing while sleeping). Too much body fat may also increase the risk for developing heart disease, diabetes, and severe obesity later in life, or aggravate existing health problems such as high blood cholesterol. Therefore, gaining weight simply to add heft is not recommended for reasons of both performance and health.

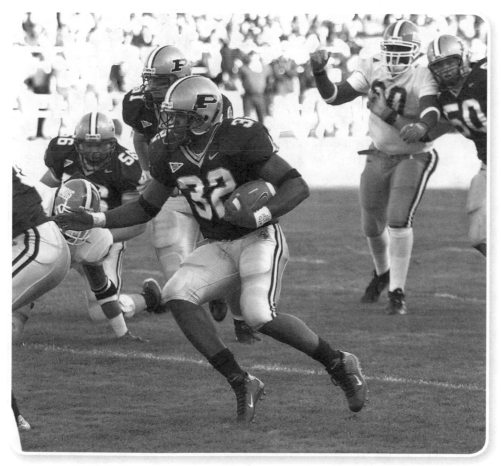

The body-composition goals of football players vary greatly depending on position. Wide receivers and running backs need a lower body-fat percentage because these positions require speed.

Size and strength are also necessary for wide receivers, running backs, and defensive backs, but running speed and agility are particularly important for these players. Defensive backs and receivers tend to have the lowest percentage of body fat among team members. Players in these positions need to be fast runners, and extra body fat becomes "dead" weight. This concept is relevant for many players in team sports such as basketball, rugby, ice hockey, soccer, and baseball, in which speed is important for excellent performance.

Football provides a great example of how players on the same team have different weight and body-composition goals. American college football players typically range from about 7 percent body fat (defensive backs) to nearly 30 percent body fat (offensive linemen). Linemen typically want to gain weight, mostly as muscle but some as fat. Running backs often want to gain weight but only as muscle, not fat. Defensive backs frequently want to increase muscle but reduce body fat.

Big, Bigger, and . . . Too Big?

Both casual observations and scientific studies suggest that athletes in contact sports have been getting bigger. For example, records from the Montreal Canadiens, a professional ice hockey team, show that compared with players in the 1920s and '30s, players in the 1980s and '90s had a similar percentage of body fat but were an average of 17 kilograms (37 pounds) heavier and 10 centimeters (4 inches) taller. Presumably, these athletes are also stronger because they have more lean body mass and better strength-training programs, but no measurements of strength were made until the 1990s. Many other sports have shown similar size progression.

Bigger, stronger, and faster are attributes that contribute to excellent athletic performance, but can athletes become too big? The increase in body weights of offensive and defensive linemen in the National Football League (NFL) has raised some cause for concern. Studies have shown that players in these positions weigh significantly more than players did in the 1970s. Most linemen on NFL rosters today weigh more than 300 pounds (136 kilograms). Although much of this weight is fat-free mass, many of these players have large amounts of abdominal fat, a risk factor for several chronic diseases. Sadly, some former NFL players suffer from serious health problems such as heart disease and diabetes.

Not surprisingly, the trend for increased size in professional linemen has had an influence on the size of collegiate and youth football players. National Collegiate Athletic Association (NCAA) Division I football players have also become bigger (as well as stronger and faster). Of great concern is the extent of overfatness in youth football, particularly among linemen, and the risk it may pose for obesity-related health problems players may experience as adults.

Getting Bigger

In the transition from high school to college, high school players often need to become "bigger" (increase their height and weight) to compete success-fully in collegiate athletics. Many college and semipro athletes also need to be "bigger" (increase their weight and muscle) to succeed as professional athletes. The way that these athletes become bigger depends on whether they have finished the adolescent growth spurt.

Athletes who are experiencing their adolescent growth spurt will gain body weight as a result of becoming taller, adding muscle mass, and increas-ing body fat. Growth occurs in all these areas because hormones associated with the adolescent growth spurt promote growth in a variety of tissues. On average, females begin their growth spurt at approximately age 10 or 11 and complete it by age 16. In contrast, males typically begin their growth spurt at age 12 or 13 and complete it by age 19. If you have not finished your growth spurt, which may not occur until college for some males, then becoming bigger will require some patience on your part.

After the growth spurt ends and adult height is reached, most athletes who want to become "bigger" typically try to build muscle mass because more muscle can result in increased strength and power and in improved speed and performance. Some underweight athletes may also want to gain a small amount of body fat.

Power Versus Endurance

Athletes are often divided into two major categories: power and endurance. At one extreme are athletes who depend only on power, such as power-lifters and shot putters. At the other extreme are those who rely primarily on endurance, such as marathon runners (figure 1.1). Most sports however, require a combination of power and endurance. For example, basketball players need short bursts of power to execute a fast break, but the length of the game requires that they also have cardiovascular endurance.

Running provides a good illustration of how the relative need for power and endurance influences weight. A 100-meter runner needs explosive power, but the distance is so short that cardiovascular endurance is not a factor. To produce the necessary explosive power, the 100-meter runner needs to have both upper- and lower-body strength. This requirement is reflected in the athlete's body composition and weight; most 100-meter runners have a large amount of muscle mass.

As the distance to be covered increases, upper- and lower-body strength remains important, but the need for endurance increases. Thus, middle dis-tance runners (400 to 3,000 meters) have less upper- and lower-body muscle mass and tend to weigh less than 100-meter runners do. Marathon runners tend to be the lightest in weight compared with other runners because a lighter body can move more efficiently than a heavier body over a long distance.

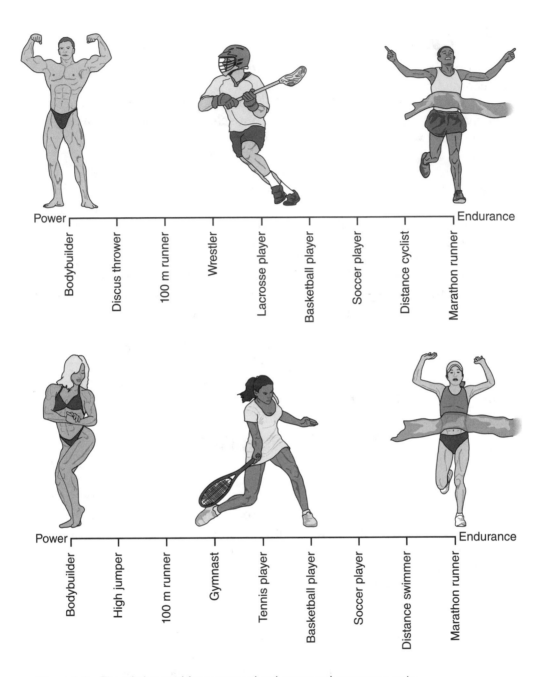

Figure 1.1 The relative need for power and endurance varies among sports.

Marathon runners must have some upper- and lower-body muscle mass to serve as a storage site for muscle fuel, but too much muscle mass is a disadvantage.

Table 1.1 provides a comparison of the height and weight of the male runners who won gold medals in the 2008 Olympics. The 100-meter runner weighs more than the other runners because of his height and the amount of muscle needed to produce explosive power. Although he may weigh a lot he is not fat! The marathon runner is the lightest. The differences in body weight and size reflect the physiological demands for power and endurance in the various running events.

TABLE 1.1

Comparisons of Height and Weight of Elite Male Runners

Name	Event	Height		Weight	
		cm	ft	kg	lb
Usain Bolt	100 m	196	6 ft 5 in.	86	190
LaShawn Merritt	400 m	191	6 ft 3 in.	84	185
Kenenisa Bekele	5,000 m	163	5 ft 4 in.	56	123
Samuel Kamau Wansiru	Marathon (26.2 mi)	163	5 ft 4 in.	51	112

Power-to-Weight Ratio

Many athletes benefit from having a high power-to-weight ratio, also referred to as relative peak power (RPP). Power can be thought of as explosive muscle strength, such as that produced by the legs of a cyclist on a tough uphill climb or by the arms of a swimmer performing the butterfly stroke. Weight refers to body weight. A high power-to-weight ratio is advantageous in many sports, and the body composition of competitive athletes reflects that fact. For example, most elite sprinters in track, swimming, and cycling have a relatively low percentage of body fat and a relatively high percentage of muscle mass for their weight. A high power-to-weight ratio is also advantageous in sports such as wrestling, gymnastics, and high jumping.

Changing the power-to-weight ratio is a primary goal for many athletes. Most athletes focus first on increasing their power by building muscle size and strength. Achieving this goal requires a well-planned resistance-training program coupled with a carefully designed diet plan to support training and the expected increase in muscle mass. Athletes can also change their power-to-weight ratio by reducing body weight in order to lose excess body fat. Unless an athlete has a large amount of excess body fat, maximizing power by building muscle mass is likely to have a more advantageous performance benefit than will minimizing body fat.

Some athletes misinterpret power-to-weight ratio to mean that attaining a very low percent body fat or low scale weight will always be beneficial. Consider the wrestler who weighs 130 pounds (59 kilograms) but decides to wrestle in the 125-pound (57-kilogram) category. He reduces his weight by 5 pounds (2.3 kilograms) and presumably has a higher power-to-weight ratio. But is it likely that he will improve his performance? The answer depends on the nature of the weight loss.

If the 5-pound (2.3-kilogram) weight loss represents excess body fat, then his power-to-weight ratio will indeed be higher and he will likely improve his performance. But if the 5-pound (2.3-kilogram) weight loss represents loss of muscle mass, then his power-to weight ratio will be lower and he will be unlikely to produce the amount of power that he did before the weight loss. These opposite outcomes highlight why athletes must learn to distinguish between weight and body composition and to monitor and reassess both during the weight-loss process.

Being a successful wrestler requires many skills, but for two opponents with equal skills, a higher body weight (relative to weight class) and a higher power-to-weight ratio confer an advantage. For this reason, athletes in weight-class sports such as wrestling, boxing, some of the martial arts, Olympic lifting and powerlifting, and lightweight rowing face considerable pressure to lose weight. If they can compete at a weight that is at the top end of a lower weight category, they may have a competitive edge over smaller opponents in that category. Many athletes, then, choose to attain a lower-than-normal body weight so that they can compete in a lower weight category.

To attain the desired qualifying weight within a short period, many athletes resort to extraordinary weight-loss methods such as short-term starvation and excessive water loss through sweating and use of diuretics. These methods can have negative effects on performance (for example, low muscle glycogen level, lower power-to-weight ratio) and health (for example, elevated body temperature). Some athletes have died while trying to cut weight rapidly when they are already dehydrated. Managing water weight is a critical topic that will be covered in chapter 8.

Sport-Specific Physical Characteristics

By now it should be clear that athletes in various sports and certain positions within team sports vary significantly in their physical characteristics. Table 1.2 groups sports together based on their physiological demands. Similarities in physical demands lead to similar body composition, weight, or nutrition-related issues for participating athletes. For example, basketball and soccer players have some commonalities because each sport requires some degree of strength, power, speed, and endurance.

Although some similarities exist, substantial differences are also present. Furthermore, significant individual differences are found between two players on the same team and even between two players who play the same position. (See chapter 2 for additional information about specific sports.) Although these general guidelines are useful, a sport assessment will help you set specific individual weight and body-composition goals. Attaining your optimal performance weight and body composition may require you to build muscle mass, decrease body fat, or both.

TABLE 1.2

Common Weight and Body-Composition Issues

Physiological demands	Sports	Weight and body-composition issues
Combat sports with weight classes	Boxing Martial arts (kickboxing, judo, taekwondo) Wrestling	▪ Weight must be certified. ▪ High power-to-weight ratio is desirable. ▪ In lower weight categories, a relatively low percent body fat is generally desirable.
Sports that emphasize appearance, aesthetics, or low body weight	Bodybuilding Figure skating Women's gymnastics Synchronized swimming Cheerleading Ballet Rhythmic gymnastics Jockeying Ski jumping	▪ Weight, body composition, or appearance is a factor in scoring. ▪ Attempts at low body weight or percent body fat may put athletes at risk for developing eating disorders.
Sports that emphasize explosive power	Sprint distances in track (50–200 m), swimming (50 m), cycling (200–500 m) Field (jumping): high, long, or triple jump, hurdles, pole vault Field (throwing): shot put, discus, hammer throw, javelin Men's gymnastics Olympic lifting Powerlifting Kayaking or canoeing (flatwater or slalom) Strength athletics (Strongman)	▪ High power-to-weight ratio is desirable. ▪ High muscularity is needed for explosive power. ▪ Relatively low percent body fat is usually desirable when body weight must be moved; percent body fat is less important when an object (for example, shot put) must be moved. ▪ Olympic lifting, Powerlifting, and Strongman competitions have weight categories.
Sports that require strength, power, speed, and endurance to various degrees	Baseball Basketball Football Ice hockey Soccer Tennis Field hockey Handball Lacrosse Racquetball Rugby Squash Volleyball	▪ Desirable weight and body composition vary depending on the sport and the position played. ▪ High muscularity and relatively low percent body fat are generally desirable if large areas of the field, rink, or court need to be covered quickly.
Sports that require a balance between power and endurance	Running: 400–3,000 m Swimming: 100–1,500 m Short-distance cycling: 1–4 km Rowing (crew) Speed skating: 500–5,000 m	▪ Weight and body composition are determined by optimal power-to-weight ratio. ▪ As distances increase, body composition tends to change from high muscularity (for explosive power) to relatively low body weight and low percent body fat (less dead weight to be carried longer distances).

(continued)

TABLE 1.2   *(continued)*

Physiological demands	Sports	Weight and body-composition issues
Sports that emphasize endurance	Distance running (>5,000 m) Distance swimming Distance cycling Duathlon Triathlon Ultradistance racing	■ Weight and body composition are determined by optimal power-to-weight ratio. ■ Relatively low body weight and low percent body fat is advantageous (less dead weight). ■ Extremely low weight or percent body fat is detrimental.
Sports that emphasize precision skills or reaction time	Golf Softball Archery Bowling	■ Strength is important. ■ Percent body fat is generally of lesser importance unless running speed is needed. ■ Golfers need some endurance if they walk the course.

Building Muscle Mass

Regardless of the sport, most athletes engage in some form of resistance training. In many cases their goal is to build muscle so that they can increase strength and power and improve performance. Although greater muscle mass is often associated with greater strength and power, for most athletes the goal should not be to gain the greatest amount of muscle mass. Rather, the goal should be to have the most effective amount of muscle mass for their sport and position.

In other words, the athlete needs the right amount of muscle because the ultimate goal is peak performance. Too little muscle can mean diminished strength or power and less than optimal performance. Too much muscle can mean reduced speed, flexibility, or agility and less than optimal performance. The whole of chapter 6 is devoted to this important issue.

Decreasing Body Fat

Lowering scale weight can be beneficial for many athletes. Because excess body fat can negatively affect speed, not carrying excess fat (dead weight) offers a potential performance advantage. *Excess* is the critical word here because some body fat is necessary for both performance and health. Reducing body fat too much can be detrimental. Essential body fat is approximately 3 percent of body mass in males and 12 to 15 percent in females.

Athletes also need to be careful about how they attain a lower scale weight because reaching a goal weight by using methods that undermine performance, such as dehydration and loss of muscle mass, is counterproductive. The potential performance advantage that may result from a lighter body weight can be offset by the disadvantages that may result from inappropriate weight-loss methods or poor timing of weight loss.

Too Much Muscle?

Dwayne (not his real name), a linebacker for an NCAA Division III college, had a high likelihood of being drafted into the NFL. During his senior year, his agent sent him to a high-level training and conditioning facility. Dwayne, a disciplined and serious athlete, understood that power and strength are essential characteristics of a successful linebacker. What Dwayne did not know was that too much of a good thing is just that—too much!

Dwayne was convinced that he needed the greatest amount of lean mass that he was able to build. He created his own nutrition plan and carefully chose high-protein, low-carbohydrate, low-fat foods plus whey protein powder, creatine, and various vitamin and mineral supplements. He was 6-feet-1-inch (185 centimeters) and weighed 260 pounds (118 kilograms), but he wanted to trim to 252 pounds (114.5 kilograms) and 9 percent body fat. By the end of his senior year Dwayne was ripped.

But Dwayne's overall caloric intake was insufficient to support his training and conditioning; his diet was too high in protein, and his nutrient intake was imbalanced. Throughout his training and his NFL evaluation, Dwayne was not prepared nutritionally. During his Pro-day evaluation, he was physically unable to complete the test exercises and had to schedule a second evaluation. Despite his poor first showing, an NFL team drafted him.

Sadly, within the first several weeks of minicamp, Dwayne was cut from the team. Despite his ultralean body and strength, he could not meet the demands of his position. The team's strength coaches felt that Dwayne's body composition was more suited to bodybuilding, rendering him inflexible, slow, and ineffective as a linebacker. Where did Dwayne go wrong? The simple answer is that he had too much muscle to meet the demands of his sport and position.

Multisport Athletes

Multisport athletes must find the right balance when it comes to their optimal weight and body composition. For example, a competitive marathon runner typically has a fairly low body weight and a low percentage of body fat. In comparison, an Ironman triathlete will likely have a higher weight and body fat percentage, even though running a marathon is part of the sport. Because of the additional demands imposed by the swim and cycling portions of the event, triathletes often find that having an extremely low percentage of body fat is not beneficial to performance.

Many high school athletes compete in more than one sport. After their season ends, some football players go immediately into wrestling. Others play basketball and then baseball. The right weight and body composition for football may not be optimal for basketball. Thus, an athlete's weight and body-composition goals can change quickly.

After the first season ends, the athlete should go through a systematic process to determine an appropriate performance weight and body composition for the next sport. End-of-season weight and body-composition measurements will need to be compared with desirable physical characteristics for athletes in the new sport. The athlete can then set goals and lay out an action plan, which includes conditioning and nutrition plans. If the time between seasons is short, making substantial changes to weight and body composition may not be realistic. Fine-tuning body composition, however, may be beneficial. The four steps to achieving optimal performance weight (assessment, goal setting, action plan, and evaluation and reassessment) provides such a process.

Identifying the Priorities for Your Sport

As discussed in chapter 1, weight and body composition are specific to the sport, the position, and the individual. To make it easier for you to understand the requirements of your sport and, ultimately, to set your personal weight and body-composition goals for improving your performance, this chapter provides position and performance characteristics for 21 sports (arranged in alphabetical order). Each sport section details typical body-composition goals and additional considerations, such as seasonal and gender information, that are unique to the sport.

You must consider *when* during the season or off-season you are going to make changes because you can undermine your performance if your timing is incorrect. For example, if you choose to trim 10 pounds (4.5 kilograms) of excess body fat and increase lean mass by 5 pounds (2.3 kilograms) before training camp begins, you will need to begin your action plan early so that it does not interfere with your preseason training and conditioning. Some factors may be sport specific, such as a requirement that your weight be certified. You must give such factors high priority. Gender considerations may be relevant. For example, body checking is allowed in male ice hockey but not in female ice hockey, a rule difference that has implications for body size, weight, and composition.

To use this chapter, begin by finding your sport and your specific position or specialty. (If you do not find your sport, choose the one that is most similar.) The performance characteristics listed are those that are highly influenced by weight and body composition. Remember, improved performance is the ultimate goal. After you set your weight and body-composition goals and priorities according to your sport and position (see chapter 4), you need to develop a specific and personalized action plan to achieve them. Once you have progressed through the chapters in part II of this book and developed your own goals, strategies, and action plan, you can incorporate the detailed meal plans for building muscle, losing fat, or simultaneously doing both found in chapters 10, 11, and 12 into your action plan. The relevant meal plan chapter is indicated for each of the sports presented in this chapter.

Baseball

Optimal weight and body composition depend primarily on the position played, the player's offensive role (for example, high batting average, power hitting), and the need for running speed.

SEASONAL FOCUS

- Make major changes to body composition and weight in the off-season.
- Fine-tune body composition and weight in the preseason.
- Maintain body composition and weight during the season.
- Avoid rapid weight loss during spring training camp because dehydration is likely to be the cause.

ADDITIONAL CONSIDERATIONS

- Making a successful transition between competition levels (high school and college; college and professional) usually requires an increase in size, strength, and speed.
- At all levels, infielders and outfielders tend to have a lower percentage of body fat than pitchers and catchers do.
- Frequent travel and late-night eating can lead to poor nutrient intake and weight gain.

Position characteristics	Performance characteristics	Body-composition goals	Meal plan
Infielder: Hits for contact Speed on base paths	Lateral speed and agility Baserunning speed	Increase muscle for strength Decrease excess body fat to increase speed Excess muscle or fat will decrease speed and agility	Chapter 12
Infielder: Hits for power	Lateral speed and agility Power hitting	Increase muscle to improve power Decrease excess body fat to increase speed Too much muscle will decrease speed and agility	Chapter 12
Outfielder: Hits for contact Speed on base paths	Short sprint and baserunning speed	Increase muscle and decrease excess body fat to increase short sprint speed Excess muscle or fat will decrease speed	Chapter 12
Outfielder: Hits for power	Short sprint speed Power hitting	Increase muscle to improve power	Chapter 10
Catcher: Hits for power	Explosive power to stand from squat Stamina Power hitting	Increase muscle to improve explosive power Excess fat may decrease stamina	Chapter 10
Pitcher: May or may not hit	Arm strength Stamina	Must set individual goals Body composition of lesser influence compared with other positions	Choose chapter 10, 11, or 12 based on individual goals

Basketball

Basketball requires size, strength, power, and speed as well as excellent aerobic conditioning. Optimal weight and body composition depend on the position played.

SEASONAL FOCUS

- Make major changes to body composition and weight in the off-season, at least three months before the season starts.
- Maintain body composition and weight during the season.
- Avoid rapid weight loss during training camp because dehydration is likely to be the cause.
- Training and performance decline with dehydration; do not confuse water weight loss with fat weight loss.

ADDITIONAL CONSIDERATIONS

- Making a successful transition between competition levels (high school and college; college and professional) usually requires an increase in size, strength, and speed.
- To stand out at any level, you must have sufficient size, strength, power, speed, and cardiovascular endurance relative to your opponents.
- Cardiovascular endurance and speed often improve when excess body fat is lost. Reducing body fat may be the top priority for recreational players.

Position characteristics	Performance characteristics	Body-composition goals	Meal plan
Point guard: Quick reflexes and court speed Height and size of lesser importance	Speed Agility Cardiovascular endurance	Increase some muscle for strength Decrease excess body fat to increase speed and endurance	Chapter 12
Shooting guard: Court speed Size and strength to take frequent shots and play perimeter defense	Speed Mobility Strength Cardiovascular endurance	Increase muscle for size and strength Decrease excess body fat to increase speed, mobility, and endurance	Chapter 12
Small forward: Quick reflexes and speed to cut to the basket	Speed Agility Cardiovascular endurance	Decrease excess body fat to increase speed and endurance Increase some muscle for strength	Chapter 11 or 12
Power forward: Height, size, strength, and mobility for rebounding and posting up	Strength Speed Mobility Cardiovascular endurance	Increase muscle for size and strength Decrease excess body fat to increase mobility and conditioning	Chapter 12
Center: Height and size but less mobility Strength to score and rebound	Strength Cardiovascular endurance	Increase muscle for strength Excess fat will decrease mobility and speed	Chapter 11 or 12

Bodybuilding

The sport of bodybuilding is subjectively judged on muscle size, definition, and proportionality, posing, charisma, and overall appearance. The goal is to have maximum muscle size and a low percent body fat.

SEASONAL FOCUS

- Working backward from the contest date, determine the number of weeks needed for each phase.
- Carefully plan diet and training details for each phase.
- Cutting weight by way of rapid and large water weight loss is physically and mentally difficult and potentially dangerous.
- Reducing body water to enhance muscle appearance is potentially dangerous.
- After a contest, muscle size and appearance decrease and weight and body-fat increase.

ADDITIONAL CONSIDERATIONS

- Natural bodybuilding competitions ban steroids and diuretics, resulting in more emphasis on diet and training techniques.
- A long-term energy deficit (low caloric intake and high caloric expenditure) can cause hormonal disruptions and menstrual irregularities.
- Mental and physical rest and recovery are needed after each contest.
- The amount of muscle that can be built varies according to gender and genetic predisposition.
- The use of some supplements to enhance body build can pose serious health risks.

Contest preparation phase	Conditioning strategy	Body-composition goals	Meal plan
Muscle building	Greater muscle size through diet and resistance training	Substantially increase muscle, although small increase in body fat may result	Chapter 10
Muscle gain while losing fat (about 10 to 12 weeks before contest)	Greater muscle size through diet and resistance training Aerobic exercise for fat loss	Decrease excess body fat Gain or maintain muscle to the extent possible	Chapter 12
Cutting weight (about 1 week before contest)	Maximize and accentuate musculature Minimize body fat	Decrease percent body fat to low level	Chapter 11

Cheerleading (Females)

The sport of cheerleading involves cheer, gymnastic, and dance routines that are subjectively judged. Cheerleaders require a strong but aesthetically pleasing body and good cardiovascular endurance to perform continuously for 2 1/2 minutes.

SEASONAL FOCUS

- Make body-composition changes slowly to prevent interference with year-round training and competitions.
- Avoid rapid weight loss because dehydration is likely to be the cause.
- Training and performance decline with dehydration; do not confuse water weight loss with fat weight loss.

ADDITIONAL CONSIDERATIONS

- A long-term energy deficit (low caloric intake and high caloric expenditure) can cause hormonal disruptions and menstrual irregularities.
- A realistic goal for a lightweight female who wants to build muscle mass is an increase of about 1 1/3 to 3 pounds (0.6 to 1.4 kilograms) of muscle per month.
- Large, simultaneous changes in weight and body composition may not be realistic. A feasible goal may be in the range of a 1- to 2-pound (0.45- to 0.9-kilogram) gain in muscle and a 2- to 4-pound (0.9- to 1.8-kilogram) loss of body fat per month.
- The ability to attain a low percent body fat varies based on body build and genetic predisposition to leanness.

Precompetition training phase	Primary focus of each phase	Body-composition goals	Meal plan
Muscle building	Greater muscle size and strength	Increase muscle	Chapter 10
Muscle gain while losing fat	Greater muscle size and strength Improved cardiovascular endurance	Decrease excess body fat Gain or maintain muscle to the extent possible	Chapter 12
Precompetition sculpting	Lean and fit appearance No excess body fat	Decrease percent body fat to relatively low level	Chapter 11

Cycling

Cycling is a diverse sport that includes track sprints that last only seconds, road races that occur over many days, and competitions that require cyclists to negotiate difficult terrain with natural and manmade hazards. Cyclists need both lower- and upper-body strength for speed, power, and handling of the bicycle, but excess body fat is not advantageous.

SEASONAL FOCUS

- Make major changes to body composition and weight in the off-season (for example, winter for road racing).
- Maintain body composition and weight during the season; high-volume training makes weight maintenance difficult.

ADDITIONAL CONSIDERATIONS

- Typically, building muscle is the primary focus because adding muscle increases power and improves performance to a greater extent than losing body fat does. Competitive cyclists typically have a low percent body fat because of rigorous training and multiday races.
- Multiday road racers need to allow enough time to recover from grueling events and may need to gain a small amount of fat before rigorous training begins again.

Specialty	Performance characteristics	Body-composition goals	Meal plan
Sprinting (track)	Strength for explosive power and sprint speed	Increase muscle Decrease excess body fat	Chapter 12
Criterium (~5 km short course)	Sprint speed and cardiovascular endurance	Increase muscle Decrease excess body fat	Chapter 12
Single-day road racing	Strength and endurance	Increase muscle and decrease excess body fat to increase speed Excess muscle or fat will decrease speed	Chapter 12
Multiday road racing (for example, Tour de France)	Strength and ultraendurance	Increase muscle and decrease excess body fat to increase speed Excess body weight is a disadvantage	Chapter 12
Mountain biking	Strength for explosive power and sprint speed Upper-body strength for bike handling	Increase muscle	Chapter 10
BMX (bicycle motocross)	Strength for explosive power and sprint speed Upper-body strength for bike handling	Increase muscle	Chapter 10

Figure Skating (Females)

Figure skating is also known as artistic skating because it combines athleticism with artistry. The athletic demands of the sport require well-developed lower-body musculature, but female figure skaters are also expected to be thin.

SEASONAL FOCUS

- Make body-composition changes slowly to prevent interference with year-round training and competitions.
- Avoid rapid weight loss because dehydration is likely to be the cause.

ADDITIONAL CONSIDERATIONS

- Skaters may set unrealistically low weight goals to offset the TV effect (people may appear 10 pounds [4.5 kilograms] heavier on TV).
- Revealing clothing increases expectations for thinness.
- The drive for thinness and perfection may be a risk factor for eating disorders.
- A long-term energy deficit (low caloric intake and high caloric expenditure) can cause hormonal disruptions and menstrual irregularities.
- To prevent health problems, calculate a minimum scale weight (see pages 66-67).
- Large, simultaneous changes in weight and body composition may not be realistic. A feasible goal may be in the range of a 1- to 2-pound (0.45- to 0.9-kilogram) gain in muscle and a 2- to 4-pound (0.9- to 1.8-kilogram) loss of body fat per month.
- The ability to attain a low percent body fat varies based on genetic predisposition to leanness.

Precompetition training phase	Primary focus of each phase	Body-composition goals	Meal plan
Muscle building	Greater muscle size and strength	Increase muscle	Chapter 10
Muscle gain while losing fat	Greater muscle size and strength Improved cardiovascular endurance	Decrease excess body fat Gain or maintain muscle to the extent possible	Chapter 12
Precompetition sculpting	Lean and fit appearance No excess body fat	Decrease percent body fat to relatively low level	Chapter 11

Football

Most football players are large bodied; the position played determines the relative need to be lean.

SEASONAL FOCUS

■ Make major changes to body composition and weight in the off-season.

■ Maintain body composition and weight during the season.

■ Avoid rapid weight loss during training camp because dehydration is likely to be the cause.

ADDITIONAL CONSIDERATIONS

■ Making a successful transition between competition levels (high school and college; college and professional) usually requires an increase in size, strength, and speed.

■ Sufficient size, strength, power, speed, and cardiovascular endurance are needed to match up well with opponents.

■ Receivers and defensive backs are leanest, linemen have the most body fat, and quarterbacks and linebackers tend to fall in between.

Position characteristics	Performance characteristics	Body-composition goals	Meal plan
Offensive lineman: Large body build	Strength Big and strong relative to opponent Power	Increase muscle for strength Some excess body fat is acceptable but too much is detrimental Usually has highest percent body fat on the team	Chapter 11 or 12
Running back: Compact, muscular build	Explosive power and speed Strength Agility Endurance	Increase muscle for size, explosive power, and strength Decrease excess body fat to increase explosive speed	Chapter 12
Receiver: Lean and muscular build	Speed Strength Cardiovascular endurance Jumping Ability	Decrease body fat to increase speed and conditioning Increase muscle for strength and size	Chapter 12
Quarterback: Height Arm strength	Sufficient speed, strength, and cardiovascular endurance Mobility	Varies Increase muscle for size and strength Decrease excess body fat to increase speed and conditioning	Chapter 10, 11, or 12
Defensive lineman: Large body build	Strength Power Big and strong relative to opponent	Increase muscle for strength Some excess body fat is acceptable but too much is detrimental	Chapter 11 or 12
Linebacker: Large, muscular build	Sufficient strength, speed, and cardiovascular endurance Mobility Agility	Increase muscle for strength Excess body fat will decrease mobility and speed	Chapter 11 or 12
Defensive back: Muscular build	Sufficient strength, speed, and cardiovascular endurance Jumping ability	Increase muscle for strength Excess body fat will decrease speed	Chapter 11 or 12

Gymnastics (Women)

Women's gymnastics requires strength, power, flexibility, and aerobic conditioning as well as a visually appealing body. Based on current aesthetic standards, the ultimate goal for many competitors is maximum muscle strength, minimum muscle size, and a thin appearance.

SEASONAL FOCUS

■ Make body-composition changes slowly to prevent interference with year-round training and competitions.

■ Avoid rapid weight loss because dehydration is likely to be the cause.

ADDITIONAL CONSIDERATIONS

■ A high percentage of lean body mass, low percent body fat, and low body weight are technical advantages for rotational moves.

■ Low body weight is currently an aesthetic advantage.

■ The drive for thinness and perfection may be a risk factor for eating disorders.

■ A long-term energy deficit (low caloric intake and high caloric expenditure) can cause hormonal disruptions and menstrual irregularities and increase the risk of stress fractures and injury.

■ To prevent health problems, calculate a minimum scale weight (see pages 66-67).

■ When comparing weight or body composition with the characteristics of the previous year, account for growth. As a rule, for each 1-inch (2.5-centimeter) increase in height expect a 5-pound (2.3-kilogram) increase in weight.

■ A realistic outcome is a 1- to 2-pound (0.45- to 0.9-kilogram) gain in muscle and 2- to 4-pound (0.9- to 1.8-kilogram) loss of body fat per month.

■ The ability to attain a low percent body fat varies based on genetic predisposition to leanness.

Precompetition training phase	Primary focus of each phase	Body-composition goals	Meal plan
Muscle building	Greater muscle size and strength	Increase muscle	Chapter 10
Muscle gain while losing fat	Greater muscle size and strength Improved cardiovascular endurance	Decrease excess body fat Gain or maintain muscle to the extent possible	Chapter 12
Precompetition sculpting	Thin appearance No excess body fat	Decrease percent body fat to relatively low level	Chapter 11

Hockey (Ice Hockey)

Ice hockey is a full-contact sport that requires size, strength, power, and skating speed as well as excellent aerobic endurance. Professional players today are taller and heavier (because of increased muscle mass) than they were in the past.

SEASONAL FOCUS

- Make major changes to body composition and weight in the off-season, at least three months before the season starts.
- Maintain body composition and weight during the season; high-volume training makes weight maintenance difficult.

ADDITIONAL CONSIDERATIONS

- Making a successful transition between competition levels (high school, college or club, and professional) usually requires an increase in size, strength, power, skate speed, and cardiovascular endurance to match up well with opponents.
- Adult male hockey players must be large bodied because body checking is legal.
- Body checking is illegal in women's hockey so body size is not as great a factor.
- Typically, building muscle is more likely to improve performance than losing body fat is.
- Cardiovascular endurance often improves when excess fat is lost. Reducing fat may be the top priority for recreational players.

Position characteristics	Performance characteristics	Body-composition goals	Meal plan
Power forward: Big and strong	Size (for body checking) Strength Speed Cardiovascular endurance	Increase muscle for size and strength Decrease excess body fat to increase speed and conditioning	Chapter 11 or 12
Center: Covers ice, wins face-offs, distributes puck	Speed Strength (esp. upper body) Agility Cardiovascular endurance	Increase muscle for strength and size Decrease excess body fat to increase speed, agility, and conditioning	Chapter 11 or 12
Winger: Intercepts passes, body checks	Speed Strength Cardiovascular endurance	Increase muscle for strength and size Decrease excess body fat to increase speed and conditioning	Chapter 11 or 12
Defender: Blocks	Speed Mobility Strength Cardiovascular endurance	Increase muscle for size and strength Decrease excess body fat to increase speed, mobility, and conditioning	Chapter 11 or 12
Goaltender: Reacts quickly to prevent scoring	Size Mobility Strength Quick reflexes	Increase muscle for size and strength Excess fat will decrease mobility	Chapter 11 or 12

Lacrosse

Men's lacrosse is a contact sport that requires strength, power, speed, and endurance. Women's lacrosse has less physical contact and two additional midfielders; thus, the women's game tends to be faster than the men's game. Optimal weight and body composition depend on the position played.

SEASONAL FOCUS

■ Make major changes to body composition and weight in the off-season.
■ Maintain body composition and weight during the season.

ADDITIONAL CONSIDERATIONS

■ Sufficient size, strength, power, speed, and cardiovascular endurance are needed to match up well with opponents and complement teammates.
■ Body composition and weight vary depending on the relative need for strength (more muscular, heavier) and endurance (less muscular, lighter).
■ Size is an advantage for men because of the physical contact of the men's game.
■ Size is less of an advantage for women because contact is limited; speed and endurance are highly valued because the women's game is faster.
■ Athletes in positions that favor speed and endurance tend to have a relatively low percent body fat.

Position characteristics	Performance characteristics	Body-composition goals	Meal plan
Attacker: Goal scorer	Speed Endurance Quick reflexes	Increase muscle for strength Decrease excess body fat to increase speed	Chapter 12
Midfielder: Gains and keeps possession of the ball Covers the entire field	Endurance Speed Strength	Increase muscle for strength and size Decrease body fat to increase speed and conditioning	Chapter 12
Defender: Prevents goals from being scored	Sprint speed Strength	Increase muscle for strength and size Excess fat will decrease speed, endurance, and mobility	Chapter 10, 11, or 12
Goalkeeper: Reacts quickly to prevent scoring Covers small area in front of the goal	Larger bodied (tall and heavier) Quick reflexes Strength	Increase muscle for strength and size Excess fat will decrease mobility	Chapter 10 or 11

Martial Arts

The martial arts are combat sports in which the goal is to defeat the opponent. Although the many disciplines vary significantly, the martial arts typically involve striking or grappling. Competitors are categorized by gender and weight.

SEASONAL FOCUS

■ Make body-composition changes slowly to prevent interference with year-round training and competitions.

ADDITIONAL CONSIDERATIONS

■ Sufficient size, strength, power, speed, and cardiovascular endurance are needed to match up well with opponents.

■ The largest competitor in a weight class is considered to have an advantage, so competitors are under pressure to compete in a lower weight category.

■ Some athletes use a short-term strategy that involves losing body fat in the week before weigh-in and gaining body fat in the days after competition. Athletes usually have difficulty achieving the lower weight when they use this strategy repeatedly.

■ Cutting weight by way of rapid and large water weight loss is physically and mentally difficult, dangerous, and potentially fatal.

■ The dangers associated with dehydration as a weight-loss method include elevated body temperature, which can be fatal.

Specialty	Performance characteristics	Body-composition goals	Meal plan
Judo	Strength Some explosive power Balance Flexibility Stamina	Increase muscle for strength and power	Chapter 10
Kickboxing	Strength Explosive power Cardiovascular endurance Balance Flexibility Stamina	Increase muscle for strength and power Decrease excess body fat to increase speed and conditioning	Chapter 12
Taekwondo	Explosive leg strength and power Cardiovascular endurance Balance Flexibility Stamina	Increase muscle for strength and power Decrease excess body fat to increase speed and conditioning	Chapter 12
Making or cutting weight		Goal is to lose enough weight (body fat or water) to certify weight but maintain muscle mass and strength	Chapter 11

Powerlifting

Powerlifting measures strength in the squat, bench press, and deadlift. Competitors are categorized by gender, age, and weight. Skeletal proportions, specifically bone length and breadth, tend to be similar among the top competitors in each weight class.

SEASONAL FOCUS

■ Powerlifters may try to build muscle mass at any time during the season.

■ Because weight classes are broad many competitors qualify easily, but some will need to make weight before weight certification.

ADDITIONAL CONSIDERATIONS

■ Being the largest competitor in a weight class is considered an advantage.

■ Powerlifters focus on building muscle mass, but an increase in body fat often occurs in the process because of excessive caloric intake.

■ Too much body fat is generally not a performance issue but excessive abdominal fat may predispose a person to future health problems.

■ A large body mass (weight) for height can contribute to joint problems.

■ Some lifters use a short-term strategy that involves losing body fat in the week before weigh-in and gaining body fat in the days after competition. Athletes usually have difficulty achieving the lower weight when they use this strategy repeatedly throughout the season.

■ Cutting weight by way of rapid and large water weight loss is physically and mentally difficult, dangerous, and potentially fatal.

■ The dangers associated with dehydration as a weight-loss method include elevated body temperature, which can be fatal.

Weight class	Performance characteristics	Body-composition goals	Meal plan
Lightweight and medium weight	Strength Explosive power	Increase muscle for strength and power Excess body fat acceptable as long as weight-class requirement is met	Chapter 10
Heavyweight: Large body mass (weight), girth, and body fat	Large bodied Strength Explosive power	Increase muscle for strength and power Excess body fat acceptable as long as weight-class requirement is met	Chapter 10
Superheavyweight: Very large body mass (weight), girth, and body fat	Large bodied Strength Explosive power	Increase muscle for strength and power Excess body fat acceptable but may create medical problems	Chapter 10 or 11
Making or cutting weight		Goal is to lose enough weight (body fat or water) to certify weight but maintain muscle mass and strength	Chapter 11

Rugby (Union)

Optimal weight and body composition depend on the position played. As rugby union has become more competitive, the fitness and conditioning levels of all players have increased.

SEASONAL FOCUS

■ Make major changes to body composition and weight in the off-season.

■ Maintain body composition and weight during the season.

ADDITIONAL CONSIDERATIONS

■ Successful players fall within a large range of percent body fat, so optimal percent body fat cannot be defined for any position.

■ Players in positions that require more strength and power are less concerned about the amount of body fat that they have as long as they have enough muscle mass.

■ Reducing excess body fat may improve cardiovascular endurance, speed, and agility.

■ For those who play more than one position, body-composition goals are a hybrid of those required for the various positions.

Position characteristics	Performance characteristics	Body-composition goals	Meal plan
Prop and hooker: Gains and keeps possession of the ball	Large bodied (height and weight) Strength Limited speed	Increase muscle for strength Some excess body fat acceptable	Chapter 10
Lock: All-around athletic skills	Height Strength Speed Endurance	Increase muscle for strength Decrease excess body fat to increase explosive speed	Chapter 12
Flanker: Gains and keeps possession of the ball	Large bodied (height and weight) Strength Speed	Increase muscle for strength and size Decrease body fat to increase speed and conditioning	Chapter 12
Number eight: All-around athletic skills	Large bodied (height and weight) Sufficient speed, strength, and endurance	Increase muscle for strength and size Decrease body fat to increase speed and conditioning	Chapter 12
Scrum-half: Exceptional ball-handling skills	Size less important Agility Quick reflexes	Varies based on the individual	Chapter 10, 11, or 12
Fly-half and wing: Fast runners Wings often score	Speed Cardiovascular endurance Agility Lateral movement	Increase muscle for strength Excess body fat will decrease mobility and speed	Chapter 11 or 12
Centre and fullback: Tackling Kicking	Large bodied (height and weight) Strength	Increase muscle for strength Some excess body fat acceptable	Chapter 10

Running (All Distances; Track and Field: Track Events)

The goal of competitive running is to cover the distance in the shortest time possible. The optimal weight and body composition depend on the distance covered and the relative need for power and endurance.

SEASONAL FOCUS

- Make major changes to body composition and weight in the off-season.
- Fine-tune body composition and weight in the preseason.
- Maintain body composition and weight during the season.

ADDITIONAL CONSIDERATIONS

- As the level of competition increases (high school to college to professional or elite recreational), competitors generally need to fine-tune body composition and weight.
- Most elite runners have a relatively low percent body fat because extra fat is dead weight.
- Sprinters tend to have a large amount of muscle mass to generate the power needed to run short distances quickly.
- Beyond sprint distances, excessive muscle becomes a disadvantage because body mass (weight) increases.
- Distance runners who have excess body fat may find that losing some fat improves performance, but having too little body fat can be detrimental to performance and health.
- The drive for thinness and perfection may be a risk factor for eating disorders, particularly for distance runners.
- A long-term energy deficit (low caloric intake and high caloric expenditure) can cause hormonal disruptions and menstrual irregularities and increase risk of stress fractures and injury.
- To prevent health problems, calculate a minimum scale weight (see pages 66-67).
- The ability to attain a very low percent body fat varies based on genetic predisposition to leanness; very low percent body fat can also be difficult to maintain.

Specialty	Performance characteristics	Body-composition goals	Meal plan
Sprints—100 m, 200 m, and 400 m	Strength for explosive power and sprint speed	Increase upper- and lower-body muscle mass Decrease excess body fat	Chapter 12
Middle distances—800 m, 1,500 m, mile, and 3,000 m	Sprint speed and some endurance	Increase muscle somewhat Decrease excess body fat Excess muscle or fat will decrease speed	Chapter 12
Long distances—5,000 m, 10,000 m, half-marathon (13 mi)	Endurance	Low body weight is advantageous Excess muscle or fat will decrease speed	Chapter 11 or 12
Marathon (26.2 mi)	Ultraendurance	Low body weight is advantageous Excess muscle or fat will decrease speed	Chapter 11 or 12

Soccer

Soccer is a limited-contact sport whose positions require various degrees of strength, power, speed, and endurance.

SEASONAL FOCUS

- Make major changes to body composition and weight in the off-season.
- Maintain body composition and weight during the season.

ADDITIONAL CONSIDERATIONS

- Competitors need sufficient size, strength, power, speed, and cardiovascular endurance to match up well with opponents and complement teammates.
- Body composition and weight vary depending on the relative need for strength (more muscular, heavier) and endurance (less muscular, lighter).
- There is no correct percentage of body fat based on position played.
- Excess body fat negatively affects speed and endurance and may limit playing time.
- Athletes in positions that favor speed and endurance tend to have a relatively low percentage of body fat.

Position characteristics	Performance characteristics	Body-composition goals	Meal plan
Forward: Playmaker and goal scorer	Height Speed Endurance	Increase muscle for strength Low percent body fat for speed, endurance, and mobility Decrease excess body fat to increase speed	Chapter 12
Midfielder: Ball control and accurate passing	Strength Speed Endurance	Increase muscle for strength and size Decrease body fat to increase speed and conditioning	Chapter 12
Defender: Prevents goals from being scored Ball control and accurate passing	Strength Speed Endurance	Excess fat will decrease speed, endurance, and mobility Varies based on relative need for strength (more muscular, heavier) and endurance (less muscular, lighter)	Chapter 10, 11, or 12
Goalkeeper: Fast reaction time	Height Strength Agility Quick reflexes Jumping ability	Increase muscle for size and strength Excess fat will decrease mobility	Chapter 10, 11, or 12

Softball (Women's Fast Pitch)

Optimal weight and body composition depend on the position played and expected contributions to scoring (short- or long-ball hitter, base stealing).

SEASONAL FOCUS

- Make major changes to body composition and weight in the off-season.
- Fine-tune body composition and weight in the preseason.
- Maintain body composition and weight during the season.
- Avoid rapid weight loss during training camp because dehydration is likely to be the cause.

ADDITIONAL CONSIDERATIONS

- Better fitness and conditioning is expected now than in the past.
- With the exception of the pitcher, most softball players do not expend much energy over the course of the game or practice sessions. Some players struggle to avoid gaining weight as body fat.
- Some players have a body type that favors fat deposition. For them, reducing body fat will be a slow process.

Position characteristics	Performance characteristics	Body-composition goals	Meal plan
Infielder: Hits to get on base Speed on base paths	Lateral speed, agility, and quick reflexes Baserunning speed	Some increase in muscle for strength Decrease excess body fat to increase speed Excess muscle or fat will decrease speed and agility	Chapter 10 or 12
Infielder: Hits for power	Lateral speed, agility, and quick reflexes Power hitting	Increase muscle to improve strength and power	Chapter 10
Outfielder: Hits to get on base Speed on base paths	Short sprint speed for fielding and base running	Increase muscle and decrease excess body fat to increase short sprint speed Excess muscle or fat will decrease speed	Chapter 10, 11, or 12
Outfield: Hits for power	Short sprint speed for fielding Power hitting	Increase muscle to improve strength and power	Chapter 10
Catcher	Explosive power to stand from squat Stamina Power hitting	Increase muscle to improve explosive power Excess fat may decrease stamina	Chapter 10, 11, or 12
Pitcher (windmill motion)	Arm strength Stamina	Must set individual goals	Choose chapter 10, 11, or 12 based on individual goals

Swimming

The goal of competitive swimming is to cover the distance in the shortest time possible. The optimal weight and body composition depend on the distance covered and the relative need for power and endurance.

SEASONAL FOCUS

- Make major changes to body composition and weight in the off-season.
- Fine-tune body composition and weight in the preseason.
- Maintain body composition and weight during the season; high-volume training makes weight maintenance difficult.

ADDITIONAL CONSIDERATIONS

- As the level of competition increases (high school to college to elite), athletes generally need to fine-tune body composition and weight. Finding the proper balance between the amount of muscle and body fat needed for optimal performance typically requires some trial and error.
- Swimmers are typically not ultralean because that body composition would be a performance disadvantage. Body fat improves buoyancy.
- Swimmers generally have a higher percent body fat when compared with runners and cyclists who cover an equivalent distance.
- Distance swimmers who have excess body fat may find that losing some fat improves performance, but having too little body fat can be detrimental to performance and health.
- Revealing clothing may increase expectations for thinness.
- The drive for thinness and perfection may be a risk factor for eating disorders.
- A long-term energy deficit (low caloric intake and high caloric expenditure) can cause hormonal disruptions and menstrual irregularities.

Specialty	Performance characteristics	Body-composition goals	Meal plan
Sprint—50 m and 100 m	Strength for explosive power and sprint speed	Increase muscle Decrease excess body fat	Chapter 12
Middle distance—200 m and 400 m	Sprint speed and some endurance	Increase muscle Decrease excess body fat Excess muscle or fat will decrease speed	Chapter 12
Distance—800 m and 1,500 m	Endurance	Excess muscle or fat will decrease speed	Chapter 11 or 12
Long distance—greater than 1,500 m	Endurance	Excess muscle or fat will decrease speed	Chapter 11 or 12
Open-water long-distance swimming (for example, English Channel)	Ultraendurance	Increase muscle Higher level of body fat may be advantageous	Chapter 10

Tennis

Tennis is played at various intensities and durations from casual games to the professional level. To stand out at any level, you must have sufficient size, strength, power, speed, and cardiovascular endurance to match up with your opponents.

SEASONAL FOCUS

- Professional and recreational players should make body-composition changes slowly to prevent interference with year-round training and competitions.
- Collegiate players should make major changes to body composition and weight in the off-season and maintain those characteristics during the season.

ADDITIONAL CONSIDERATIONS

- Professional tennis players are typically taller and weigh more today than players did in the past.
- Successful collegiate and professional players fall within a large range of percent body fat. Optimal percent body fat cannot be defined for the sport.
- Reducing excess body fat may help improve cardiovascular endurance, speed, mobility, endurance, and stamina, especially at the recreational level.

Level of competition	Performance characteristics	Body-composition goals	Meal plan
Professional	Sufficient height and weight Strength Cardiovascular endurance Mobility	Some increase in muscle for strength and body size Decrease excess body fat to increase speed Excess muscle or fat will decrease speed and mobility	Chapter 10 or 12
Collegiate	Strength Cardiovascular endurance Mobility	Some increase in muscle for strength Decrease excess body fat to increase speed Excess muscle or fat will decrease speed and mobility	Chapter 10 or 12
Recreational (2.5–5.0 ranking)	As ranking increases, cardiovascular endurance is a greater influence At lower rankings, skill is the greatest influence	Varies depending on the individual Excess body fat may decrease speed, mobility, endurance, and stamina	Chapter 10, 11, or 12

Track and Field: Field Events

Field events consist of individual throwing or jumping events or a combination of these events. Body composition is largely influenced by the need to move either an object or the body through space.

SEASONAL FOCUS

- Throwers are less concerned about body composition and may try to build muscle mass at any time, including during the season.
- Jumpers, decathletes, and heptathletes should make major changes to body composition and weight in the off-season.
- Decathletes and heptathletes should fine-tune body composition and weight during the preseason; these changes may be aided by a return to high-volume training.

ADDITIONAL CONSIDERATIONS

- Making a successful transition between competition levels (high school, college, and professional) may require an increase in size, strength, power, speed, and endurance.
- Throwers focus on building muscle mass, which increases strength and body weight. Increases in body weight because of increased body fat may be advantageous.
- For throwers, too much body fat is generally not a performance issue, but excessive abdominal fat may predispose a person to future health problems.
- Jumpers generally try to build or maintain muscle mass, but they should achieve and maintain a fairly low percent body fat to avoid carrying dead weight.
- Decathletes and heptathletes should not be too muscular nor have excessive body fat because of the range of events required. Such athletes generally excel in events well suited for their natural body composition, whether it favors speed or endurance.

Position characteristics	Performance characteristics	Body-composition goals	Meal plan
Throwers—shot put, hammer, javelin, discus	Large bodied Strength Explosive power	Increase muscle for strength and power Some excess body fat acceptable because it adds body weight	Chapter 10
Jumpers—high jump, pole vault, long jump, triple jump	Sprint speed Explosive power	Increase muscle for strength and power Excess body fat is dead weight	Chapter 12
Decathlon (men) and heptathlon (women): combination of sprint and middle-distance running, throwing, and jumping	Speed Strength Endurance	Increase muscle for strength and speed Decrease excess body fat to increase speed and endurance Excess muscle or fat is a disadvantage	Chapter 12

Triathlon

Triathlon is an ultraendurance sport for professionals and amateurs that consists of swimming, cycling, and running. Distances vary according to the event.

SEASONAL FOCUS

- Professionals should make body-composition changes slowly to prevent interference with year-round training and competitions.
- Amateurs should make major changes to body composition and weight several months before the triathlon.

ADDITIONAL CONSIDERATIONS

- Professional triathletes tend to have a relatively low percent body fat but not as low as that of long-distance runners or cyclists.
- An extremely low percent body fat is a disadvantage because body fat provides buoyancy for swimming and a source of calories for ultraendurance training.
- Reducing excess body fat may help improve endurance, speed, and stamina, especially at the amateur level.
- Many amateurs choose to compete in a triathlon because they want to increase their fitness and conditioning and lose body fat, typical consequences of months of high-volume training.
- Body composition is less important if the amateur's goal is simply to finish.

Level of competition	Performance characteristics	Body-composition goals	Meal plan
Professional, Ironman—2.4 mi (3.8 km) open water swim, 112 mi (180 km) cycle, and 26.2 mi run (marathon)	Ultraendurance Speed Strength	Some increase in muscle for strength Decrease excess body fat to increase speed Excess muscle or fat will decrease endurance and speed Too little body fat affects ultraendurance capability	Chapter 12
Professional, Olympic length—1.5 km (.93 mi) swim, 40 km (24.8 mi) cycle, and 10 km (6.2 mi) run	Endurance Speed Strength	Some increase in muscle for strength Decrease excess body fat to increase speed Excess muscle or fat will decrease endurance and speed	Chapter 12
Amateur, Ironman, or Olympic length	Endurance Speed Strength	Varies depending on the individual Excess body fat may decrease endurance and speed	Chapter 10, 11, or 12

Wrestling

Freestyle wrestling is a hand-to-hand combat sport that has weight classes based on age and gender. With two opponents of equal skill, a higher body weight and a higher power-to-weight ratio are likely to offer a performance advantage. In practice, this means that a physical and possibly a psychological benefit may result from achieving the maximum weight of a lower weight category.

SEASONAL FOCUS

- Make major changes to body composition and weight in the off-season.
- When comparing weight or body composition to the characteristics of the previous year, account for growth. As a rule, for each 1-inch (2.5-centimeter) increase in height expect a 5-pound (2.3-kilogram) increase in weight.
- Collegiate and high school regulations include the establishment of a minimum weight class before the season begins, a higher minimum weight class if weight is gained during the season, and limiting competitors to a weight class that is one higher than their established minimum.
- High school wrestlers must meet minimum body-fat percentages (7 percent for males, 12 percent for females), and the maximum amount of weight that can be lost per week is mandated.
- These regulations emphasize building muscle mass and losing body fat slowly.

ADDITIONAL CONSIDERATIONS

- Sufficient size, strength, power, stamina, and skill are needed to match up well with opponents.
- Being the largest competitor in a weight class is considered an advantage, so wrestlers are under pressure to compete in a lower weight category.
- Some wrestlers use a short-term strategy for achieving a certain scale weight before weigh-in that involves dehydration and semistarvation. Athletes usually have difficulty achieving the lower weight when they use this strategy repeatedly throughout the season.
- Cutting weight by way of rapid and large water weight loss close to the time of weigh-in is physically and mentally difficult, dangerous, and potentially fatal.
- The dangers associated with dehydration as a weight-loss method include elevated body temperature, which can be fatal.

Wrestling, *continued*

Weight class	Performance characteristics	Body-composition goals	Meal plan
Lighter weight wrestlers	Strength Explosive power Cardiovascular endurance Balance Flexibility Quick reflexes	Increase muscle for strength and power May have body type that does not gain large amounts of muscle quickly	Chapter 10
Middle-weight wrestlers	Strength Explosive power Cardiovascular endurance Balance Flexibility Quick reflexes	Increase muscle for strength and power Decrease excess body fat to increase power-to-weight ratio	Chapter 12
Heavyweight wrestlers	Large bodied Strength Explosive power Cardiovascular endurance Balance Flexibility Quick reflexes	Increase muscle for strength and power May have body type that gains large amount of fat quickly	Chapter 11
Making weight		Goal is to lose enough weight (body fat or water) to certify weight but maintain muscle mass and strength	Chapter 11

Analyzing Your Body, Assessing Your Weight

Assessment creates a picture of where you are. It involves physical measurements such as height, weight, somatotype (body build), girth, and body composition, as well as physiological assessments including current state of health, energy (calorie) intake, and energy (calorie) expenditure. Your current dietary intake needs to be accurately recorded so that energy and nutrient consumption can be evaluated. Assessing physical activity and metabolic rate are ways to determine usual energy expenditure. All assessments must be as complete and accurate as possible.

You use this information as the basis for setting goals and developing your action plan. Assessment allows you to

- compare your body to current standards in your sport,
- set achievable and realistic goals based on your body type,
- avoid setting ill-conceived goals that undermine performance,
- estimate the magnitude of changes that you need to make,
- establish a realistic time frame for meeting your goals, and
- objectively evaluate your progress and adjust your plan as needed.

Because each assessment method provides specific information, you should seek to obtain as many of the measurements mentioned that are available and affordable. You will use these measurements to establish goals that are well matched for your sport and the position that you play. You will also use some of the measurements as a basis for comparison later to determine whether your weight management strategies are working as planned. Assessment will help you set weight and body-composition goals that can improve your performance. Remeasurement is an unbiased way to determine whether you are making progress toward your goals. Some of the assessments take time, but you will find that this time is well spent.

Physical Assessments

Height, weight, body build, and girth measurements are physical assessments that are relatively easy to measure. These measurements give you general information about your physical size and a basis for comparison with other athletes in your sport. Weight and girth are also useful in evaluating changes over time.

Height and Weight

Height (stature) and weight (body mass) are two easily performed measurements used to determine an optimal performance weight. Your weight and height can be compared with the typical range for your sport or position. Weight-class sports have regulated weight categories that athletes must conform to in order to compete. In many sports, successful athletes customarily fall into certain weight ranges.

Optimal weight is relative to height. An optimal weight at 6 feet (183 centimeters) tall may be overweight at 5 feet, 9 inches (175 centimeters). Although you surely know your approximate height, you should have an accurate measurement because many formulas include height as a factor. A simple way to obtain an accurate measurement is to stand barefoot on a hard surface and against a wall with your heels, buttocks, shoulders, and head touching the wall while you are looking straight ahead. Stand as straight and tall as possible while someone places a ruler on your head at a 90-degree angle to the wall and marks the wall at the underside of the ruler. The distance from the floor to the mark on the wall is your height. Measurements made at home are reasonably accurate, but the most accurate measurements are those that use a measurement board permanently attached to the wall (such as at a doctor's office) because carpet, baseboards, and old measuring tapes that have been stretched can all introduce measurement error.

Weight is easily measured with a properly calibrated scale. For greatest accuracy, weigh yourself in the morning at the same time, with the least amount of clothing on, before eating and after urinating, and using the same scale each time. One weight measurement does not tell the whole story. Your weight can be an indication of several things, including hydration status. Normal fluid fluctuations cause weight to vary slightly from day to day and even from morning to evening. Daily weight measurements can help you estimate how much fluid you lose during exercise and serve as a guideline for rehydration.

But to assess changes in body composition that are not fluid related, you should take a series of weekly weight measurements to obtain a picture of your usual weight range over time. Weight is best referred to as a range rather than a single number. Scale weight is too imprecise to rely on just one number. A weight range prevents misinterpreting small but beneficial changes in muscle or fat tissues.

Fat and Muscle Weight Differences

You may have heard people say that muscle weighs more than fat. What they mean is that muscle is more dense than fat. One pound (0.45 kilogram) of muscle is so compact that it takes up only one-third of the space that 1 pound of fat does. As an example, think of raisins and grapes. Twenty raisins would fit in a tablespoon, but a 1-cup measuring cup would be needed to hold 20 grapes. Because of the difference in density between muscle and fat, those who start an exercise program often find that weight initially goes up because they are building muscle but they also find that they are reducing girth because they are losing fat.

You may be wondering—should I gain weight or lose weight? The answer depends on your body-composition goals. If your goal is to increase only muscle mass, then your weight will go up. If you lose only body fat, then your weight will go down. If you increase muscle mass more than you decrease body fat, then your weight will go up. If the weight of muscle mass that you gain is equal to the weight of body fat that you lose, then your weight will be the same. The preceding examples point out one of the major limitations of scale weight—it cannot be used to determine body composition. For many athletes in training, an increase in body weight is positive because it reflects an increase in muscle mass.

You can use the Track Your Progress form from appendix B to record your current age, height, and weight and to track your progress over time. After you have set your goals and objectives and have developed and instituted your strategies, you will need these baseline data to monitor your progress.

Somatotype (Body Build)

Somatotyping is a way to categorize athletes visually. The terms used are ectomorph (thin), mesomorph (muscular), and endomorph (stocky) and are illustrated in figure 3.1. Ectomorphs are described as having a slight build with small amounts of fat and muscle. Endomorphs have a stocky build and a tendency to gain body fat easily, especially in the abdomen. Mesomorphs are muscular and typically do not gain large amounts of body fat.

Although people frequently have features of more than one somatotype, having an idea of your predominant somatotype category is important in choosing a sport or position that is best suited to your body type and for setting realistic body-composition goals. A person built with a predominantly ectomorphic somatotype may be better suited to be a long-distance runner, wide receiver, or figure skater rather than a football lineman, powerlifter, or shot putter, activities that favor an endomorphic body type. Knowing your predominant somatotype helps in setting realistic goals for building muscle mass and understanding the sculpting potential of your body.

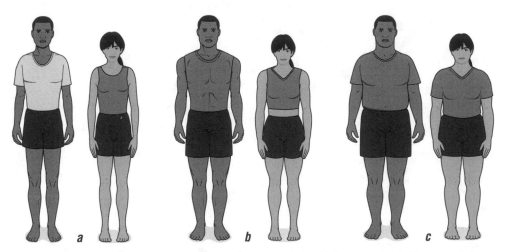

Figure 3.1 The three general body types are ectomorph (*a:* thin), mesomorph (*b:* muscular), and endomorph (*c:* stocky).

Reprinted, by permission, from National Strength and Conditioning Association, 2008, *Essentials of strength training and conditioning*, 3rd ed. (Champaign, IL: Human Kinetics), 145.

An unbiased professional can provide the most accurate assessment of your somatotype, but self-assessment is possible if you have an accurate body image. Each somatotype has specific characteristics. By looking at yourself in a mirror you can get a general idea of your somatotype. Note that you may have characteristics of more than one type.

Girth Measurements

Girth measurements can be used to track changes over time in body size and proportionality. A flexible metal tape is used to measure the girth (circumference) of body parts at six sites, typically waist, hips, thighs, calves, arms, and chest. These measurements are among the easiest to obtain, and most can be self-administered. Although girth measurements are not a direct measure of the percentage of body fat or lean mass, they can help you track changes in body composition. Loss of body fat often results in a decrease in the girth of the waist, hips, and thighs if excess fat is stored in those areas. An increase in muscle mass can result in a considerable increase in the circumference of the arms, thighs, and calves. A change in a girth measurement can be a good motivator to continue with your current action plan.

Body Composition

Height, weight, somatotype, and girth are easy to measure with reasonably good accuracy, but an accurate body-composition measurement is more difficult to obtain. An assessment of body composition must be part of a comprehensive plan to achieve optimal performance weight. Total body weight is only part of the picture. The composition of that weight is the other, and often more important, part. Unless your body composition is measured, you will not know whether the weight that you are losing is body fat or whether you are maintaining, increasing, or decreasing muscle mass.

Discussion of body composition requires definition of some terms. The body is composed of four major components: fat, muscle, bone, and water. A simple way to discuss optimal performance weight and body composition is to divide the body into the two general components of fat and lean. Body fat exists as essential fat or storage fat. Essential fat, the fat contained in organs (for example, heart) and tissues (for example, nervous system), is required for normal physiologic functioning, including reproduction.

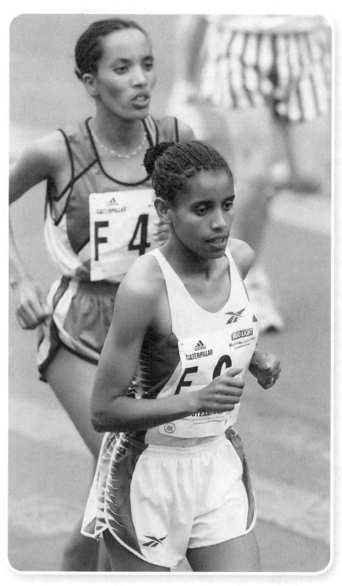

An athlete's predominant somatotype influences the sports and positions that are best suited to her. Distance running, for example, favors ectomorphic body types over endomorphs.

Essential fat represents approximately 3 percent of body mass in males and 12 to 15 percent in females. Storage fat is deposited primarily beneath the skin in adipose tissue, but some is found around vital organs where it serves as a protective cushion.

Fat-free mass and *lean mass* are terms used to describe the lean portion of the body. Although these terms are often used interchangeably, they are not the same. Fat-free mass refers only to the lean tissues of the body and does not include any fat stores. Lean mass refers to muscle, bone, water, and essential fat stores. For practical purposes, lean mass is the term most often used in discussions of body composition, but it does not refer solely to muscle mass.

As shown in table 3.1, several methods are used to measure body composition. Some methods are more accurate and consistently reproducible than others, but all methods produce some error. Each method has advantages and disadvantages. Your choice of assessment method will depend on several factors, including availability, cost, and need for precision. Availability is especially important because you need to choose one method and stick with it. Choose the most accurate measure that is practical, available, affordable, and that you can use repeatedly to measure your progress. The results obtained from the various body-composition assessment methods should *not* be compared. Comparing underwater weighing with skinfold measurements is like comparing apples and oranges.

To determine which method of body-composition analysis is best for you, a good rule is to choose the most reliable method of body-composition assessment that is affordable and reasonably accessible. To find out what is available in your area, contact a sports dietitian, exercise physiologist, or certified strength and conditioning professional. Check with local universities, training and conditioning facilities, health and fitness clubs, or sports medicine practices. Staff at stores that sell high-quality fitness equipment may be able to direct you to a reliable testing center. After you choose a method, you may look to manufacturers of body-composition equipment to locate local testing centers. Manufacturers' Web sites may include a tab for locating a qualified testing professional in your area.

After your body composition is assessed, use the Track Your Progress form in appendix B to record the results. Reassessing body composition is an important part of step 4 (evaluation and reassessment) of the four steps to achieving optimal performance weight. Body composition is typically reassessed about every six weeks because the body needs time to change in response to exercise and changes in caloric intake (see the evaluation and reassessment sections in chapters 6 and 7 for more information).

Physiological Assessments

Physiological assessments, such as a physical exam and measurement of metabolic rate, nutrient intake, exercise output to quantify energy expenditure, and relative peak power give you specific information about yourself.

TABLE 3.1

Methods for Assessing Body Composition

Method	Accuracy*	Advantages	Disadvantages	Pretest preparation	Cost and accessibility
Dual-energy X-ray absorptiometry (DEXA or DXA)	5	Highest accuracy when compared with other methods	Expensive Limited availability	None	About $300 University research facilities and imaging centers with specialized body-composition software
Hydrostatic (underwater) weighing	4	Well-trained technicians	Water submersion Time consuming	No food or water 2–3 hours beforehand	$10–$75 but may be free if a current student University exercise physiology labs and some fitness clubs
Body plethysmography (BOD POD)	4	Quick and easy	Need compression bathing suit and cap	No food or exercise 2 hours beforehand	$40–$75 Some fitness clubs and university laboratories
Skinfold thickness	3	Fairly quick and easy	For accurate measurement, the technician must be properly trained, have experience, and use the proper equipment	None	Free or low cost Someone on staff at a school or health club may have the proper training
Bioelectrical impedance (BIA)	3	Quick and easy	For accurate measurement, pretest protocol must be followed	Must be fully hydrated No food, water, or caffeine 4 hours beforehand No moderate exercise 12 hours beforehand No alcohol 48 hours beforehand	Free to $40 Widely available at schools, health fairs, fitness clubs
Near-infrared interactance (NIR)	2	Quick and easy	Less accurate than other methods	None	Cost varies Available at some fitness clubs and training facilities

*1 = less accurate and 5 = more accurate (based on published research).

Some assessments must be precisely measured, whereas others can be estimated. In some cases assessments may require medical or metabolic tests (for example, blood analysis, peak power) because obtaining an accurate estimate is not possible. Assessments of dietary intake and physical activity depend on accurate self-recording of information. Although conducting these assessments may be time consuming, they provide valuable information for setting realistic weight and body-composition goals, and they form the basis of all measures of progress.

State of Health

One assessment that athletes may overlook unless it is required is an annual physical. Even a physically fit 20-year-old athlete may have health problems or the potential for health problems. For example, a female runner may assume that she is sluggish because she has not been getting enough sleep, but a blood test taken as part of a physical exam may reveal that she has iron deficiency anemia.

Family history may put you at risk for diseases such as diabetes or cardiovascular disease. Early detection and treatment are important to your health and fitness as well as your performance. Having a physical exam each year and before beginning a training and conditioning program is prudent.

Dietary Intake

A record of your usual dietary intake is an indispensable component of a comprehensive assessment. This dietary snapshot provides information about the amount of food (that is, calories) and nutrients consumed daily as well as the pattern of food and beverage intake throughout the day (that is, the frequency of meals and snacks). This baseline information is essential for devising a plan to change your weight and body composition.

For a representative view of usual dietary intake, you need to measure and record all that you eat and drink over a typical three-, five-, or seven-day period. Three days is considered the minimum needed, but five or seven days will give you a better picture. Physical activity is often recorded for seven consecutive days. The Food Intake Record Form in appendix B can help you with this assessment.

When recording your food intake, you should eat as usual. Do not adjust food consumption to conform to a diet that you believe you should be eating or cut back on your food intake. Food preparation methods and the addition of condiments, sauces, gravies, and salad dressings all contribute to calories and overall nutrients. Be sure to include this information. Dietary intake studies have shown that people routinely underestimate portions when recording food intake. Therefore, careful measurement and complete recording is essential to obtaining an accurate assessment. Although this process requires time and effort, it is the only way to measure your food intake precisely.

The following tips can help you record your food intake accurately:

▪ Use the same glass and cup for all beverages that you consume during the recording period, if possible. Before the recording period begins, fill the glass or cup with water and then measure the water so that you know how much the glass or cup holds. If you typically fill the glass or cup with varying amounts of fluid, mark those levels on the glass or cup and measure those amounts.

▪ For bottled or canned beverages, note the number of ounces or milliliters in the container and record the amount that you consume. For restaurant drinks, ask your server what the volume of the cup is in ounces (or milliliters), if possible. Be mindful that the server may fill your cup with more liquid throughout the meal; you need to record those amounts.

▪ When you first eat a particular food during the recording period, select the portion that you would typically eat and then measure it before eating. Second and third helpings need to be measured and recorded as well. After you have measured food that you have served yourself, use the same bowls and serving spoons each time you choose that food or a similar food.

▪ Whenever possible, use a food scale to weigh cooked, boneless portions of meats, poultry, or fish. Note the preparation method: broiled, fried, baked, grilled, boiled, sauteed, and so on. Record additions such as breading, sauces, and gravies. When eating in restaurants, ask your server for the cooked weight of the meat, fish, or poultry.

▪ Use level (not heaping) measures in measuring cups and spoons.

▪ When recording fruits and vegetables include any additions such as sauces, syrups, or other ingredients added to the food and note how the vegetables are prepared.

▪ For grain products, indicate that they are whole wheat, rye, white, oat, multigrain, and so on. For bagels, record the size in inches (centimeters) or ounces (grams). For tortillas, note the diameter.

▪ For prepared foods, read the Nutrition Facts label and be sure to note the serving size. Packages often contain more than one serving. If you eat more than the designated serving, you must adjust the nutrient and caloric information accordingly.

▪ Review the Additional Tips for Recording Food Intake page in appendix B for more information about how to record your food intake accurately.

After you complete your food intake record, you need to analyze the information that you have collected. A dietary analysis is typically done by entering daily food and beverage intake into a nutrient analysis software program. (See appendix A for a list of Web sites that have analysis programs.)

Nutrient analysis software is only as good as the database on which the program is based, so be sure to choose a program that uses the USDA Nutrient Database as its foundation. After you have entered your food intake, the program will calculate the amount of energy and nutrients contained in those foods.

These raw data are used as a baseline assessment of your usual energy and nutrient intake, which is the first step toward completing a comprehensive nutrition assessment. Nutrients are measured in grams (g), milligrams (mg), or micrograms (mcg, or μg). You may run across three measurements for energy—kilocalories (kcal), Calories (C), or calories (cal). The correct scientific and international measurement of energy is kilocalories or Calories, not calories. A calorie (lower case *c*) is a very small

Figure 3.2   Dietary Intake Assessment Results

	Energy (kcal)	Carbohydrate (g)	Protein (g)	Fat (g)
Day 1				
Day 2				
Day 3				
Day 4				
Day 5				
Day 6				
Day 7				
Daily average				

unit of measure. For example, a teaspoon of sugar has 15 kilocalories or Calories but 15,000 calories. In the United States, these terms are used interchangeably. People often read that 1 teaspoon (4 grams) of sugar has 15 calories, but this statement is not technically correct.

Use figure 3.2 to record the amount of kilocalories, carbohydrate, protein, and fat consumed each day and your average daily intake. The computer program will usually indicate whether you were deficient in any vitamins or minerals by comparing your intake to the Dietary Reference Intake (DRI). The DRI is the current standard used in the United States and Canada to judge nutrient inadequacies and excesses. You can find more information about the amount of each nutrient needed in chapter 5.

	Nutrient deficiencies (list each nutrient)	Excessive intake (list each nutrient)
Day 1		
Day 2		
Day 3		
Day 4		
Day 5		
Day 6		
Day 7		
Daily average		

Physical Activity

Of the factors that affect your daily energy requirements, physical activity is the greatest variable. It has a profound effect on your energy needs. As an athlete, the energy to fuel your conditioning, training, and performance represents a significant proportion of your total calorie needs. The types of physical activities and the duration and intensity at which you perform them will have an effect on the amount of calories and type of fuel that you burn while exercising.

To estimate the energy used daily, record all your activities each day for a typical seven-day period. You will need to record activities of daily living (for example, sitting while eating and working, sleeping) as well as any exercise performed. Note the intensity and duration of exercise. For

Figure 3.3   Physical Activity Assessment Results

	Training intensity (rest, low, moderate, high) and duration
Day 1	
Day 2	
Day 3	
Day 4	
Day 5	
Day 6	
Day 7	
Daily average	

your convenience, an Activity Record form is provided in appendix B. The process is similar to the recording of usual food intake and can be done at the same time.

After you have completed your activity records, you can calculate the calories expended for physical activity by entering them into an online calculator (see appendix A for Web sites) or the nutrient analysis program that you used to calculate the calories consumed from food. Use figure 3.3 to record your usual daily caloric expenditure and your average daily expenditure. Also note the intensity and duration of exercise. Comparing your daily food intake and energy expenditure will help you evaluate whether the amount and timing of your food intake is sufficient to support your volume of training.

	Energy output (kcal)
Day 1	
Day 2	
Day 3	
Day 4	
Day 5	
Day 6	
Day 7	
Daily average	

Certified Specialists in Sports Dietetics

This book will help you determine your best weight and body composition for optimal performance and plan a diet to build muscle or lose fat. Athletes can successfully reach their goals on their own, but you may reach a point where you want to seek specialized expertise. If so, consider using the services of a Certified Specialist in Sports Dietetics (CSSD). A CSSD is a registered dietitian with demonstrated expertise and experience in sports nutrition.

A sports dietitian will conduct a comprehensive dietary assessment using a powerful nutrient analysis program and interpret the results. A CSSD will help you view your nutrient intake in the context of your energy demands, weight management and body-composition goals, and your overall health and well-being. In addition to planning an individualized muscle-building or fat-loss diet, a sports dietitian will guide and support you along the way.

To locate a sports dietitian, log on to the Sports, Cardiovascular, and Wellness Nutrition (SCAN) Web site at www.scandpg.org; click on About SCAN; and choose Search for a SCAN Dietitian. SCAN is a dietetic practice group of the American Dietetic Association, the largest organization of food and nutrition professionals in the United States.

Metabolic Rate

Simply put, metabolic rate is the rate at which your body's engine uses energy. You can increase your metabolic rate by building muscle mass or decrease it by adhering to a starvation-type diet. Metabolic rate can be recorded at rest or during exercise. Specialized equipment is required to measure metabolic rate during exercise, so athletes commonly estimate their metabolic rate at rest.

Resting metabolic rate (RMR) is an estimate of the number of calories that the body needs to maintain its basic functions. RMR does not take into consideration the energy used during physical activity. In general, RMR accounts for approximately 75 percent of all calories expended daily by a sedentary person. It represents at least 50 percent of daily energy expenditure by most trained athletes, although there are tremendous individual variations in resting metabolic rate.

Why is knowledge of your resting metabolic rate useful? One reason is that RMR estimates the minimum amount of calories that you need to consume to provide your body with the energy for its basic physiological functions. When daily caloric intake is severely reduced, the body responds to the starvation state within a couple of days by lowering its RMR and conserving energy output. For example, if your RMR is 1,900 kilocalories daily and you decide to go on a crash diet for a week by consuming only 1,200 kilocalories daily, then your body is in a starvation state.

Studies have shown that RMR can decrease by 20 percent or more under such conditions, so in this example RMR could decline to about 1,500 kilocalories. The decline in RMR is counterproductive to weight-loss efforts (see chapter 7). Many people use RMR to make sure that they are not going on a starvation-type diet. Athletes do not perform well when they are starving, so this assessment is especially important for athletes who are trying to achieve a low weight or a low percentage of body fat.

You can estimate your resting metabolic rate in several ways. First, you can do a simple calculation to get a rough estimate. This is the quickest but least accurate method. If you have determined your body composition, you can better predict resting metabolic rate by using the Cunningham formula. The most precise estimation of RMR involves using a metabolic measurement system, but this method requires specialized equipment and trained technicians. Although obtaining a direct measurement is always more accurate than making an estimate using a simple calculation or formula, using simple methods is better than not having this important piece of assessment information.

Simple Calculation of RMR.   You can estimate your resting metabolic rate by using an online RMR calculator (see appendix A for Web sites). Another simple method is to find your weight and gender in table 3.2. These easy methods are the least accurate ways to estimate RMR.

Cunningham Formula.   The Cunningham formula is a prediction equation that is considered one of the best ways to estimate RMR for athletes because it incorporates body composition. Research shows that other formulas significantly underestimate the RMR of both male and female recreational and elite athletes. The Cunningham formula follows:

$$500 + (22 \times \text{FFM in kg}) = \text{RMR}$$

To use the Cunningham formula, you need to determine your fat-free mass (FFM) in kilograms. The first step is to convert your weight in pounds to kilograms using the following equation or table 3.3:

$$\text{Weight in lb} / 2.2 = \text{weight in kg}$$

The next step is to use your body-composition results to determine your percentage of FFM. Do this by subtracting your percentage of body fat from 100:

$$100 - \% \text{ body fat} = \% \text{ FFM}$$

Then, you can easily determine your FFM in kilograms by multiplying your percentage of FFM by your weight in kilograms:

$$\% \text{ FFM} \times \text{weight in kg} = \text{FFM in kg}$$

After you have determined your FFM, you can place this figure into the Cunningham formula to determine your RMR. As an example, table 3.4 shows how the Cunningham formula is used to calculate the RMR of a 159-pound (72.3-kilogram) male cyclist who has 12 percent body fat.

TABLE 3.2

Estimate of Resting Metabolic Rate*

Weight (lb)	Weight (kg)	RMR females (kcal/day)	RMR males (kcal/day)
100	45.5	983	1,092
110	50.0	1,080	1,200
120	54.5	1,177	1,308
130	59.1	1,277	1,418
140	63.6	1,374	1,526
150	68.2	1,473	1,637
160	72.7	1,570	1,745
170	77.3	1,670	1,855
180	81.8	1,767	1,963
190	86.4	1,866	2,074
200	91.0	1,966	2,184
210	95.5	2,063	2,292
220	100.0	2,160	2,400
240	109.1	2,357	2,618
260	118.2	2,553	2,837
280	127.3	2,750	3,055
300	136.4	2,946	3,274

* Females: weight (kg) $\times$ 0.9 kcal/kg $\times$ 24 hr; males: weight (kg) $\times$ 1.0 kcal/kg $\times$ 24 hr.

TABLE 3.3

Body Weight in Pounds and Kilograms

WEIGHT			
Pounds	Kilograms	Pounds	Kilograms
100	45.5	200	91.0
110	50.0	210	95.5
120	54.5	220	100.0
130	59.1	230	104.5
140	63.6	240	109.1
150	68.2	250	113.6
160	72.7	260	118.2
170	77.3	270	122.7
180	81.8	280	127.3
190	86.4	290	131.8

TABLE 3.4

RMR for 159-Pound (72.3-Kilogram) Cyclist With 12 Percent Body Fat

Weight (lb)	Weight (kg)	% body fat	% FFM	FFM (kg)	Cunningham formula: 500 + (22 × FFM in kg)	Predicted RMR
159	72.3	12	88	63.6 kg	500 + (22 × 63.6)	1,899 kcal

Direct Measurement of RMR. Metabolic measurement systems measure oxygen consumption at rest and use that figure to estimate RMR from a standardized formula. The simplest systems are handheld, require only a nose plug, and take only 5 to 10 minutes. Because oxygen consumption is measured directly, this estimate is more accurate than any prediction equation. A measurement of RMR using a handheld device may be available at some health and fitness clubs, training facilities, and offices of sports-related professionals.

The measurement of oxygen consumption by a handheld device is not as accurate as a full metabolic measurement system, which measures both oxygen consumption and carbon dioxide production and then calculates RMR. A full metabolic measurement system can also measure metabolic rate during exercise and the type of fuel used (carbohydrate or fat) at various exercise intensities. The availability of a full metabolic measurement system is limited by the space, technical expertise, and time required to perform the measurements. You may be able to obtain a full metabolic measurement at a university exercise physiology lab, in the office of a sports-related professional, or at a training facility. A trained technician must administer the test and interpret and apply the results.

Relative Peak Power

Relative peak power (RPP), one of many measures that can be made in the exercise physiology laboratory, is used to design and evaluate strength-training programs. One of the most widely used tests of both average and peak power of the lower body is the 30-second Wingate test. After a brief warm-up, the athlete pedals a cycle ergometer, which is set to a known resistance, as fast as possible for 30 seconds. Upper-body power can be measured using a modified Wingate test or an arm ergometer.

Peak power on the cycle ergometer is measured in the first five seconds as watts (W). Because body size and weight vary among athletes, determining relative peak power permits comparison between athletes. RPP is calculated by dividing peak power (in watts) by body mass (in kilograms), giving the athlete a way to track whether her or his power-to-weight ratio is improving.

Charting Your Course for Success

After you have completed physical and physiologic assessments, the next step is to interpret those measurements. You must determine whether your current weight and body composition are well matched to your sport and whether they support peak performance. If you want to change your weight or body composition, you need to use your assessment information to set specific goals. This chapter will help you interpret the assessment information correctly and set clear goals and objectives.

Body Composition of Well-Trained Athletes

Elite athletes in most sports fall within a particular range of percent body fat, as shown in table 4.1. The data in the table have been collected from research studies of well-trained collegiate or elite athletes and then summarized. Unfortunately, the usual body composition of trained athletes for many sports has never been studied.

Such data must be interpreted carefully. Although the information documents the percent body fat of some of the successful athletes in a sport, an athlete who achieves that range will not necessarily improve performance. The range may be a good guideline, but it is not the gospel. The ability to achieve a particular body composition depends in part on your genetic makeup and somatotype.

Target Body Composition and Weight

You now have the information that you need to compare your physical assessments with successful athletes in your sport. You can use this information to set your personal body-composition and weight goals. Choose a realistic range rather than a single percentage of body fat. Select this range by considering your specific sport and genetic predisposition.

TABLE 4.1

Estimated Body Compositions of Selected Well-Trained Athletes

Sport	Level	Position or distance	% body fat
MALES			
Baseball	College	All positions	11–17
Baseball	Professional	All positions	8.5–12
Basketball	Professional	Centers	9–20
		Forwards	7–14
		Guards	7–13
Cycling, road	Professional	Long distance	7–10
Football	College (NCAA Division I)	Defensive backs	7–14.5
		Receivers	9–16.5
		Quarterbacks	14–22
		Linebackers	12.5–23.5
		Defensive linemen	14.5–25
		Offensive linemen	18.5–28.5
Judo	National team	All weight classes	8.5–19
Rugby	Professional	All positions	9–20
Soccer	Professional and college	All positions	7.5–18
Tennis	Elite		8–18
Water polo	National team		6.5–17.5
Wrestling	College champions		6.5–16
FEMALES			
Running	Elite	Middle distance	8–16.5
		Long distance	12–18
Soccer	College	All positions	13–19
Swimming or diving	College	Middle distance or diving	17–30
	Masters	Long distance	20–34
Tennis	Elite		15–25

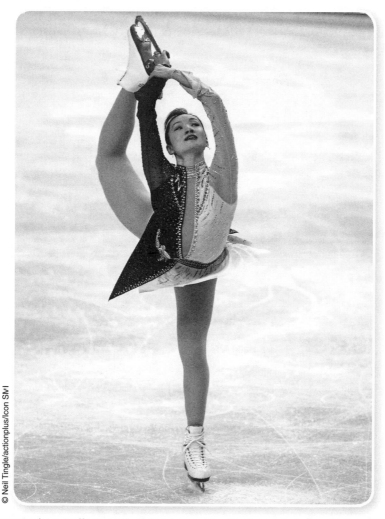

© Neil Tingle/actionplus/Icon SMI

To prevent adverse affects on their training and health, figure skaters and other athletes in low-weight sports should avoid a scale weight that is too low for their bodies.

Use Figure 4.1 on pages 64 and 65 as a starting point. For example, a male college soccer player may set a goal of 12 to 15 percent body fat, which is well within the range of most elite and collegiate players (7.5 to 18 percent). Your predominant somatotype may be useful information here because mesomorphs (muscular type) may be able to reach and maintain a lower percent body fat than endomorphs (stocky) can. The key is to choose a realistic percent body fat range for you.

In chapter 3 we discussed the importance of essential body fat. Body fat should not drop below 3 percent for males or 12 to 15 percent for females because health problems can result if percent body fat falls below those levels. Few athletes need to be this lean, and many athletes cannot safely attain and maintain such a low percentage of body fat.

Figure 4.1   Physical Assessments Comparison

Physical assessment	Personal measurements
Height	
Weight	
Somatotype	
Girth measurements	

Body composition:
   % body fat
   % lean mass	

Calculating Target Weight

Besides setting a body-composition goal, most athletes also set a weight goal. After you have determined a realistic body-composition range, you can determine a body-weight range that reflects that. The target body-weight formula that follows will help you determine your target body weight. This formula is used predominantly by athletes who want to lose body fat. The formula is an estimate that you use to establish points in a weight range, in either pounds or kilograms, that support training and peak performance. (The equation requires that you know how much fat-free mass you currently have, which is one reason that you need to measure body composition.)

Target body weight = current fat-free mass / (1 − % desired body fat)

Physical assessment	Successful athletes in your sport
Height	
Weight	
Somatotype	
Girth measurements	
Body composition: % body fat % lean mass	

As an example, consider a male collegiate soccer player who is beginning his sophomore year. He currently weighs 165 pounds (75 kilograms), has 18 percent body fat, and has 135 pounds (61.4 kilograms) of fat-free mass. After completing the assessment process he believes that he can improve his speed, cardiovascular endurance, and performance if he modestly reduces his body fat to 15 percent. By using the target body-weight formula as shown, he can determine how much body fat he needs to lose. In his case, if he loses 6 pounds (2.7 kilograms) of body fat, he will achieve his body-composition goal.

Target body weight = 135 lb / (1 − .15)
Target body weight = 135 / .85
Target body weight = 159 lb
165 lb − 159 lb = 6 lb

All simple formulas make significant assumptions and must be interpreted correctly. This target body-weight formula assumes that body composition has been measured accurately.

Take the time to calculate your target body weight now. Over the course of the year, you should plug different body-fat percentages into the formula because your body-composition goals typically change during the off-season, across training cycles, and for peak performance. The best time to lose body fat is typically in the off-season or early in the preseason. Delaying the task of changing body composition until late in the preseason or during the competitive season is often counterproductive to peak performance.

Calculating Minimum Weight

Athletes who compete in weight-class sports or sports in which low body weight is advantageous should know the minimum amount that they could safely weigh. The minimum target body-weight formula can be used to determine this weight:

> Minimum target body weight = current fat-free mass / (1 – minimum % desired body fat)

As an example, consider the case of a female bodybuilder who is new to the sport and is preparing for her first contest, which is three months away. She does a sport assessment and discovers that successful competitors are muscular and have little body fat. She currently weighs 134 pounds (60.9 kilograms) and has 20 percent body fat. Her local contest has only two weight classes: up to 125 pounds (56.8 kilograms) and over 125 pounds. She wants to compete in the lower weight category and have the lowest percentage of body fat that is healthy, which she knows is at least 12 percent for a female.

At her current body weight, she has approximately 27 pounds (12.3 kilograms) of fat (134 pounds × 20 percent) and 107 pounds (48.6 kilograms) of fat-free mass (134 pounds – 27 pounds). Assuming that she has the potential to be very lean, she could choose 12 percent as her minimum desired percent body fat. She can calculate her minimum target weight goal as follows:

> Minimum target body weight = 107 lb / 1 – .12
> Minimum target body weight = 107 lb / .88
> Minimum target body weight = 122 lb

Theoretically, this athlete could eventually weigh as little as 122 pounds (55.5 kilograms). The target body-weight formula helps her to realize that setting a goal weight lower than 122 pounds is not attainable or realistic. Note that attaining and maintaining a very low percentage of body fat is often difficult because the body is not biologically comfortable living on the edge.

Many athletes train and perform better if they have a low percentage of body fat but are not at their biological limits. Even bodybuilders, who pride themselves on attaining an extremely low percentage of body fat for competition, do not try to maintain this low level between contests. In other words, athletes have a number of different target weights to coincide with their various training and performance periods. Therefore, you should think of weight and body composition as ranges even when you are calculating a single scale weight. The hypothetical bodybuilder's weight range is 122 to 134 pounds (55.5 to 60.9 kilograms), which reflects a percent body fat range from 12 to 20 percent.

High school wrestling federations now use the minimum target bodyweight formula to establish the lowest weight class for each wrestler. Athletes in low-weight sports, such as distance running and women's gymnastics and figure skating, also use it to avoid attaining a scale weight that is too low. A body weight that is too low hinders training and performance and undermines health. For example, when energy (calorie) expenditure is consistently greater than energy intake over many months or years, an energy deficit eventually develops, which can alter metabolism, affect hormonal secretion, and, in females, disrupt menstruation. Over time, a routine energy deficit can have serious, detrimental consequences such as the female athlete triad—disordered eating, amenorrhea, and osteoporosis.

Baseline Energy Intake and Expenditure

Caloric assessment is an integral part of every plan to change weight or body composition. The estimate of your current intake and expenditure is referred to as baseline. Baseline energy (caloric) intake and output is the starting point to determine the amount of calories that you will need to build muscle or lose body fat.

If you want to lose body fat, then you must expend more calories than you consume. If you want to build muscle mass, you will likely need to eat more calories than you are currently consuming. If you want to build muscle mass and lose body fat at the same time, then you must finely tune your caloric intake on a daily basis. Specific information about caloric requirements to achieve these goals is found in part II of this book, but right now you need to determine your baseline caloric intake and expenditure so that you can set specific goals.

By comparing your dietary intake and physical activity, you can determine whether you are in energy balance, which means that you consume and expend the same amount of calories. Using the results from your dietary intake and physical activity assessments, compare your energy intake and expenditure estimates as shown in figure 4.2. (You may have recorded this information for three, five, or seven days.)

Figure 4.2   Assessing Energy Balance

	Day 1	Day 2	Day 3	Day 4
Energy intake (kcal)				
Energy output (kcal)				
Caloric difference (+ or − kcal)				

Look first at the last column, daily average, and determine whether you are in overall energy balance. For example, if your caloric intake for seven days averaged 3,000 kilocalories and you expended an average of 3,000 kilocalories, then you are in energy balance. If you consume more calories than you expend, you will experience a gain in body fat. Likewise, if you

	Day 5	Day 6	Day 7	Daily average
Energy intake (kcal)				
Energy output (kcal)				
Caloric difference (+ or − kcal)				

expend more calories than you consume, you will lose body fat and be unable to build additional muscle mass. This information will help you set specific objectives (for example, how many calories you need daily) to support your weight and body-composition goals.

You may be in energy balance over the entire seven-day period, but your intake and expenditure may not be in balance on a day-to-day basis. Many athletes find that their appetites do not keep up with energy needs when the intensity and duration of their training are high. Your dietary intake and physical activity assessments give you valuable information not only about energy but also about your eating and exercise patterns. This information will help you create an action plan to reach your specific objectives and general goals.

Examining your daily caloric intake allows you to ensure that you are not consuming too few calories. By comparing your estimated resting metabolic rate (RMR) with your daily caloric intake, you can evaluate whether you are consuming a starvation-type diet. For example, if your RMR is 1,600 kilocalories daily but your dietary assessment shows that you are only consuming 1,500 kilocalories daily, then you are essentially starving yourself. This circumstance is counterproductive to losing body fat and is at odds with any plan to build muscle mass.

Setting Goals and Objectives

Charting a course to success requires using assessment information to set goals and objectives. Then you can develop an action plan for achieving those goals. The process is not complete until you conduct an evaluation to determine whether you have achieved the initial goals. All the time and effort needed to complete the assessments now pays off because you can set personal goals and objectives. Goals can be thought of as broad, general intentions, whereas objectives are narrower, more specific. Objectives are the small steps that you take to meet your goals.

Athletes need to set at least three essential goals. One goal should be performance based. A second goal should concern weight or body composition. A third goal should be health based. You may have many goals but make sure that you have at least three goals that together address performance, weight and body composition, and health issues. These goals will help you create the right balance and keep you focused on what is important—improving performance and promoting health.

For example, look at the goals that the aforementioned female bodybuilder might set for herself (see figure 4.3). Remember that she wants to compete in the up to 125-pound (56.8-kilogram) weight category and that her contest is three months away. She sets three goals:

1. To place 10th or higher in her first contest (performance-based goal)
2. To attain a weight lower than 125 pounds (56.8 kilograms) and a body composition of about 14 percent body fat (goal pertaining to weight and body composition)
3. To continue to menstruate (health-based goal)

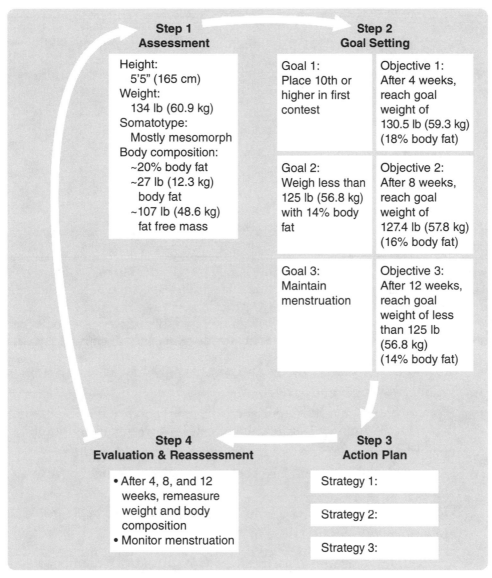

Figure 4.3 Four steps to achieving optimal performance weight for a 134-pound (60.9-kilogram) female amateur bodybuilder. (Strategy development is discussed in part II of this book.)

These goals are appropriate because she has balanced her focus on weight and body composition with a focus on performance and health. She also used her assessment information to set realistic personal goals that are attainable in her given time frame. After she set her goals, she then set some objectives, which are small steps or minigoals. To see how objectives work in practice, look again at her plan as shown in figure 4.3. To determine specific weight and body-composition objectives, she calculates target weights that she hopes to attain during the 12 weeks of training before her first contest (see table 4.2). For example, at 14 to 16 percent body fat her target body

TABLE 4.2

Weight and Body-Composition Objectives for a Female Bodybuilder

Current fat-free mass*	Current % body fat	Desired % body fat	Formula	Target body weight	Time to achieve target weight
107 lb (48.6 kg)	20	18	107 lb / (1 − .18) 48.6 kg / (1 − .18)	130.5 lb (59.3 kg)	4 weeks
107 lb (48.6 kg)	18	16	107 lb / (1 − .16) 48.6 kg / (1 − .16)	127.4 lb (57.9 kg)	4 weeks
107 lb (48.6 kg)	16	14	107 lb / (1 − .14) 48.6 kg / (1 − .14)	124.4 lb (56.5 kg)	4 weeks

*For simplicity, this example assumes that fat-free mass, such as skeletal muscle, does not change.

weight would be between 124.4 and 127.4 pounds (56.5 to 57.9 kilograms). These objectives are realistic and attainable within a specified period, increasing the likelihood of her success.

The following questions can help you begin to formulate your goals and objectives. Incorporate the answers into your goals and objectives.

- How long do I have to change my body weight and body composition?
- What is my target body-weight range?
- Is power-to-weight ratio important to my sport and position? If so, what body composition will support the greatest power-to-weight ratio?
- How much muscle mass is right for my position and my body?
- How much lean mass can I expect to gain in the time that I have available?
- How much body fat can I lose in the time that I have available?
- How many calories do I need to consume daily?

When setting goals and objectives, you should also remember to be SMART. The acronym SMART is a way of reminding athletes that goals and objectives should be specific, measurable, attainable, realistic, and time-driven.

Specific.   Perhaps the first goal you write down is "I want to improve my performance." The problem with this goal is that it is too general and broad. You must state specifically what you mean by "improve my performance." Instead, state a specific performance goal, such as "I want to decrease my mile time by 30 seconds." This specific goal embraces your general goal of improving performance and provides an objective yardstick for measuring your progress. If you are having trouble coming up with specific goals, write down your general goal and then think about what you must do to achieve it.

Measurable.   Goals need to be measurable. Simply stating, "I want to lose weight" does not give you enough information to measure progress. How much weight? What is the composition of the weight loss? To measure goals, you must be able to quantify them. An example of a measurable goal is "I want to lose 20 pounds (9 kilograms) and reduce my body fat by 3 percent." Goals need to be measurable because if you do not measure it, you cannot manage it.

Attainable.   Great athletic achievement requires great expectations. Aim high to achieve magnificent results. In aiming high, however, you must consider the realm of possibility. For instance, how likely is it that a 6-foot 3-inch (190.5-centimeter) male could be the winning jockey at the Kentucky Derby? What is the possibility that a 5-foot 2-inch (157.5-centimeter), 105-pound (47.7-kilogram) female volleyball player could make the U.S. Olympic volleyball team? Or that a 158-pound (71.8-kilogram) wrestler could make weight in the 118-pound (53.6-kilogram) weight class? Successful people stretch the limits and achieve great things, but goals and objectives must be attainable.

Realistic.   Great expectations must be doable. Deciding whether your goal is realistic is crucial to achieving success. Setting a modest yet challenging goal with a reasonable chance of success is better than establishing an over-ambitious goal that you are unlikely to achieve. Be honest with yourself. Only you know whether a goal is challenging enough or too challenging. You will find that achieving a challenging goal has a domino effect that leads to more successes. Each success builds on the next.

Many people are unrealistic about how fast they can lose body fat. An overweight athlete may say, "I'm going to lose 20 pounds (9 kilograms) in two weeks," an overambitious goal that offers little chance of success. Because the goal is unrealistic, the athlete may use drastic, even dangerous, methods in an attempt to achieve it. When the athlete fails to reach this goal, judging the effort as a failure would be easy. A realistic goal would be to lose 2 to 4 pounds (0.9 to 1.8 kilograms) in two weeks. A small loss of body fat is a success that can motivate a person to continue to lose weight. Each small weekly weight loss leads to more success until the 20 pounds (9 kilograms) are lost.

Time Driven.   Time is an important component of goal setting because time creates a sense of urgency. "We have 5 minutes to score a winning touchdown." "I need to swim the 100-meter freestyle in less than 50 seconds to qualify." In the world of sport, speed and endurance are measured by time. Even pain tolerance is measured in time. Establishing a time frame for achieving your goals helps you maintain momentum and allows you to gauge your progress. If progress slows, you can take measures to get back on track.

Commit in Writing

Write down your goals to make them clear, concrete, and real. Written goals help keep you focused on what you want to achieve. Post the goals where you can see them every day to motivate you and keep you on track. Written goals are easier to evaluate because they are concrete. You need to evaluate your goals at regular intervals to see whether you are moving forward or taking a slight detour. Regular evaluation is nearly impossible if you do not write down your goals.

Establishing a Time Frame

The general time frame for accomplishing your goals may already be set for you based on the start of your competition season. The specific time frame for achieving your goals before competition is largely determined by when you begin your action plan. Moderate, steady change is not only more sustainable but also more supportive of optimal performance. Of course, in some instances a slow and steady approach will not allow you to meet your goals. If you participate in a weight-class sport, your goal may be to drop some weight just before weigh-in. In this case, following the safest methods for making weight is crucial to protecting both performance and health.

If you are serious about success, then you need to understand that achieving your optimal weight range and body composition takes time. Not surprisingly, weight and body-composition goals need attention during the off-season and during the preseason training and conditioning periods. The off-season is the time to start, especially if you need to lose a large amount of body fat. Beginning early gives you a chance to plan for steady progress, which is more effective and long lasting than instituting a drastic change. During preseason training and conditioning, athletes often focus on fine-tuning their body weight or composition so that they can enter the competition period fully prepared for peak performance.

Unfortunately, some athletes give little thought to their best performance weight until right before the competition season begins, a time when it is most difficult to achieve weight goals. During the competitive season, the main focus is on performance. Trying to change weight substantially is often detrimental to performance. No matter where you have set your weight or body-composition goals, timing is important. Use the recommendations and time frames in table 4.3 as guidelines to make sure that you have ample time to achieve your goals.

TABLE 4.3

Guidelines for Speed of Weight Loss or Gain

Goal	Recommended amount to gain or lose per week	Time needed for a 10 lb (4.5 kg) change
Build muscle	0.5–1 lb (0.23 kg–0.45 kg) gain per week	About 10 to 20 weeks (2 1/2 to 5 months)
Lose fat	1–2 lb (0.45–0.9 kg) loss per week	About 5 to 10 weeks

Evaluating and Reassessing Goals

Goals that are SMART form the basis of effective strategies for your action plan. You may have already discovered that setting goals is relatively easy. The harder part is changing your current behavior to achieve those goals. After you develop an individualized plan, track your progress, evaluate whether you have met your goals, and make adjustments if needed. Weight and body-composition goals are measurable, so initial and follow-up measurements will be a critically important yardstick for measuring your progress.

When plans appear to be going well, evaluation is often omitted, but do not make this mistake. Remember, evaluation is step 4 in the four steps to achieving optimal performance weight and it requires reassessment of many of the original assessment measures. Evaluation provides the basis for measuring progress and adjusting plans as needed. If your strategies are cumbersome or your progress is too slow or too fast, you can adjust parts of your plan to get back on track. At times, you may even need to adjust your goals.

Let's return to the example of the bodybuilder. As shown in figure 4.3, this athlete will remeasure weight and body composition at 4, 8, and 12 weeks so that she can evaluate and monitor progress. She will also be monitoring her monthly menstruation. Depending on the outcome of the evaluation, she may need to adjust her goals and objectives. For example, if she stops menstruating, she may have failed to consume enough calories to maintain her hormonal balance. Or she may find that 14 percent body fat is too low and that she is developing harmful eating behaviors in an attempt to remain at that percentage of body fat. In either case, she is endangering her health. She would benefit from adjusting her goals and objectives.

You can use the Track Your Progress form (appendix B) to record initial and follow-up assessment measurements. Post this form in a visible place or keep it in your journal where you can continue record keeping and monitor how well you are meeting your goals. Record keeping provides the data needed for evaluation and keeps you focused and engaged in the process. Research has shown that the very act of recording has benefits, so you are wise to keep accurate and up-to-date records.

After you achieve your initial goals, you will need to set different goals that support staying on top. In other words, you need to maintain your successes. Changing behaviors so that they become habits takes time and repetition. Resetting your metabolic engine does not happen overnight. For these reasons, charting your course takes time, attention, and effort and will likely involve some adjustments along the way.

Strategies for Achieving Your Target Weight

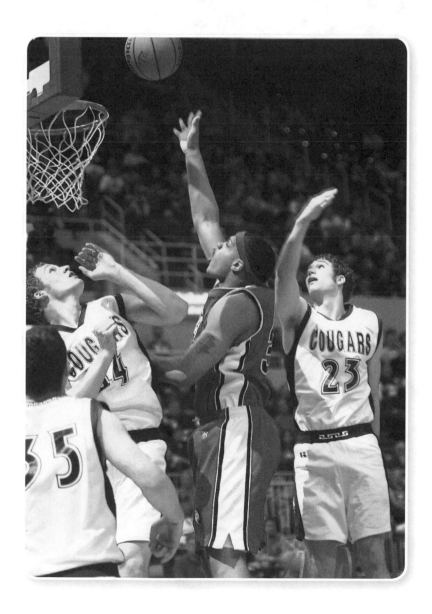

5

Building a Solid Nutritional Base

Two major goals for any serious athlete are to maximize training and conditioning and to improve performance. To achieve these goals, an individualized training and conditioning program is essential. Adhering to such a program requires proper nutritional support. You can compare this concept to what you would do to build a house; you need a well-designed architectural plan (your training and conditioning program) as well as the best possible building materials (your nutrition plan).

Food provides the energy and nutrients that you need to train and perform. Food also resupplies the nutrients that you deplete during training, which you must restore before the next training session. You need the right nutrients to build muscle, fuel physical activity, and maintain health; food is the vehicle for obtaining those nutrients. This chapter provides an overview of the nutrients that athletes need and the foods that contain them.

Essential Nutrients

The body requires more than 40 essential nutrients. These nutrients can be divided into seven groups: carbohydrate, protein, fat, vitamins, minerals, water, and fiber. Carbohydrate, protein, and fat are known as macronutrients, whereas vitamins and minerals are micronutrients because they are needed in smaller quantities. Essential nutrients provide energy, promote growth and development, and regulate body functions as shown in table 5.1. For peak performance and optimum health you must consume adequate amounts of all the essential nutrients. Without adequate amounts your body will be unable to function, train, or perform optimally.

Sports nutrition recommendations are usually based on kilograms of body weight. If you know your weight in pounds, simply divide the number by 2.2 to convert your weight to kilograms. The conversions are shown for you in table 3.3 on page 58.

TABLE 5.1

Three Main Functions of Essential Nutrients

Provide energy	Promote growth and development	Regulate body functions
Carbohydrate	Protein	Protein
Fat	Fat	Fat
Protein	Vitamins	Vitamins
	Minerals	Minerals
	Water	Water
		Fiber

Note: Although it provides energy (calories), alcohol is not an essential nutrient.

Energy Requirements

Energy, defined as the ability to do work, is measured in Calories, or kilocalories. As noted earlier, in the United States the term "calories" is used to indicate the number of Calories or kilocalories. Athletes need enough calories to have the energy to train but not too many because excess calories, regardless of the source, are stored as body fat. You must adjust calorie intake when you want to change body composition. For example, to build muscle, you need to make sure that you are consuming enough calories, but when you need to lose body fat, you need to make sure that you are not consuming too many. The difference between enough and too much is relatively small, so energy intake for athletes is usually discussed in 100-kilocalorie increments (for example, 2,000 kilocalories, 2,100 kilocalories, 2,200 kilocalories).

Energy (or calories) comes from four food sources: carbohydrate, protein, fat, and alcohol. Carbohydrate and protein yield 4 kilocalories per gram, whereas fat provides 9 kilocalories per gram, more than twice as many calories for the same weight (see table 5.2). Alcohol contributes 7 kilocalories per gram. Fat and alcohol are often described as being calorie dense because they contain many more calories per gram than carbohydrate or protein does.

TABLE 5.2

Sources of Calories

Calorie source	Calories per gram
Carbohydrate	4
Protein	4
Fat	9
Alcohol	7

Alcohol and an Athlete's Diet

You may wonder if, and how, alcohol fits into the athlete's diet. Alcoholic beverages can significantly raise calorie intake but do not contribute vitamins and minerals needed for muscle growth, performance, and health. Additionally, such beverages can unfavorably alter the carbohydrate, protein, and fat balance of your meal plan and undermine your efforts to change body composition. Alcohol calories are either excess calories or they displace needed carbohydrate, protein, or fat.

When calorie needs are high and nutrient intake is adequate, an occasional alcoholic beverage will not pose a problem. When attempting to build muscle or lose weight, every calorie counts, so athletes are wise to curtail alcohol intake until they meet weight and body-composition goals. Additionally, athletes need to refrain from drinking alcohol if it is prohibited by their team or by the rules of the governing body for their sport. Alcohol has many effects on the body and on performance:

- Acts as a depressant
- Interferes with nerve transmission and brain communication
- Impairs reaction time, coordination, and balance
- Compromises speed, strength, and endurance
- Competes with products needed for normal energy production
- Cannot be used by skeletal muscle for energy
- Increases the risk of dehydration because of its diuretic effect
- Impairs the ability of the body to regulate temperature
- Increases the need for B vitamins
- Results in a greater production of fat, which can accumulate in the liver

How many calories you need each day depends on several factors, but a major factor is the amount of energy expended each day by physical activity. Physical activity includes bodily movement during the day (for example, walking) and exercise (for example, vigorous body movement). The type, intensity, and duration of exercise will affect the number of calories that you need. Table 5.3 lists guidelines for estimating daily energy expenditure based on body weight in kilograms. People tend to overestimate the intensity and duration of their exercise, so be sure to choose a realistic figure.

Female athletes generally need 35 to 40 kilocalories per kilogram of body weight daily, unless they are engaged in rigorous endurance training. Male athletes generally need 38 to 45 kilocalories per kilogram of body weight daily except for rigorously trained endurance athletes. For example, a 154-pound (70-kilogram) female athlete would likely require 2,450 to 2,800 kilocalories daily. After you have chosen an estimate for kilocalories per kilogram, you can calculate your estimated daily caloric needs.

TABLE 5.3

Estimated Daily Caloric Needs for Male and Female Athletes

Activity level	Examples of activity level	Examples of athletes	Estimated daily caloric need (kcal/kg)	
			Females	Males
Sedentary (little physical activity)	Sitting or standing with little activity, for example, desk or computer work, light housekeeping, TV, video games, and so on	During recovery from injury	30	31
Moderate-intensity exercise 3–5 days/ week or low-intensity and short-duration training daily	Playing recreational tennis (singles) 1–1 1/2 hr every other day Practicing baseball, softball, or golf 2 1/2 hr daily, 5 days/week	Baseball players Softball players Golfers Recreational tennis players	35	38
Training several hours daily, 5 days/week	Swimming 6,000–10,000 m/day plus some resistance training Doing conditioning and skills training for 2–3 hr/day	Swimmers Soccer players	37	41
Rigorous training on a near daily basis	Performing resistance exercise for 10 to 15 hr/week to maintain well-developed muscle mass Swimming 7,000–17,000 m/day and resistance training 3 days/week	Bodybuilders (maintenance phase) College and professional basketball and American football players Elite swimmers Rugby players	38–40	45
	Training for a triathlon	Non-elite triathletes	41	51.5
Extremely rigorous training	Running 15 mi (24 km)/day or the equivalent	Elite runners, distance cyclists, or triathletes	50 or more	60 or more

Although a general estimate is helpful, you should recognize that the intensity and duration of training varies considerably based on the time of year. The athlete's year is often divided into four periods—off-season, early preseason, late preseason, and the competitive season. For more precise planning, you need to estimate your daily caloric needs for each of these periods. Your caloric needs are typically lowest in the off-season because the intensity and duration of your training are low. As your volume of training increases, you expend more calories. Estimates for each period of training will be important for determining the amount of calories that you need each day to change weight and body composition, especially because body-composition and weight goals typically change during the off-season, across training cycles, and for peak performance.

Carbohydrate

The primary function of carbohydrate is to provide energy. One of the most important parts of every athlete's diet is sufficient carbohydrate daily because all athletes need to restore the glycogen that has been depleted by exercise. Without proper replacement of glycogen, athletes can experience early fatigue, inability to train properly on consecutive days, or poor performance.

Carbohydrate is found in the body primarily as glycogen in muscle and liver cells and as glucose in the blood. When muscle is being exercised it prefers to obtain its carbohydrate from muscle glycogen rather than from liver glycogen or from the blood. Muscle can use the glycogen in its cells efficiently because it does not need to be transported. The brain and the nervous system also need a ready supply of carbohydrate from the blood. When the diet is insufficient in carbohydrate, mental and emotional functioning can be impaired, possibly resulting in fatigue, irritability, reduced concentration, sleeplessness, and depression.

Athletes in training generally need 5 to 8 grams of carbohydrate per kilogram of body weight daily, about 50 to 60 percent of total calories (see table 5.4). Studies have shown that carbohydrate intake should be at least 5 grams per kilogram daily to replenish the muscle glycogen used during light training. But this amount is not enough for athletes who train rigorously on consecutive days. A carbohydrate intake of 8 grams per kilogram daily is likely needed to restore glycogen levels in strength athletes, athletes in stop-and-go sports such as soccer and basketball, and endurance athletes after rigorous training. Endurance and ultraendurance athletes, such as triathletes, may need more than 8 grams per kilogram daily to restore muscle glycogen over weeks and months of rigorous distance training, but most athletes do not need such high levels of carbohydrate daily.

TABLE 5.4

Estimated Daily Carbohydrate Needs

Activity level	Carbohydrate needs (g/kg)
Minimum needed by athletes to resynthesize muscle glycogen after light training	5
Athletes in moderate training	6–7
Athletes in heavy training (rigorous strength training, stop-and-go athletes, and endurance athletes)	8
Endurance and ultraendurance athletes in lengthy rigorous training periods; athletes who are carbohydrate loading	8 or more

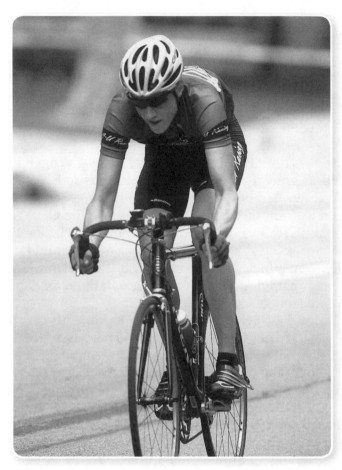

Athletes such as cyclists who train rigorously day after day need to consume enough carbohydrate to replenish their muscle glycogen.

Carbohydrate is the primary source of energy for moderate- and high-intensity exercise (the intensity at which most athletes train), so failing to restore muscle glycogen on a daily basis will undermine training and peak performance. Adequate carbohydrate intake also spares protein from being used as energy, which as you will see in the protein section beginning on page 86, contributes to the ability of your body to build tissue and regulate other processes.

Simple and Complex Carbohydrate

Carbohydrate is found in foods that contain sugars and starches. Carbohydrate occurs in complex and simple forms. Complex carbohydrate is found in whole grains (for example, wheat), beans (for example, white beans), and tubers (for example, potatoes and yams) that have been minimally processed and contain vitamins, minerals, and fiber. Simple carbohydrate occurs naturally in milk, fruits, and vegetables, as well as in sugar (for example, white sugar) and grains that have been highly processed.

Distinctions must be made among the foods with simple carbohydrate because their nutrient content varies markedly. Milk, fruits, and vegetables provide many nutrients in addition to carbohydrate. Milk contains protein, several vitamins, and the mineral calcium. Fruits and vegetables contain fiber and a wide variety of vitamins, such as vitamins A and C. In contrast, white sugar does not provide vitamins, minerals, or fiber. The simple carbohydrate category also includes highly processed complex carbohydrate (also known as refined carbohydrate or sweetened grains). In the processing, many of the nutrients and much of the fiber are removed, greatly reducing the nutrient content. Additionally, sugar or fat are added, which adds calories.

Another difference among foods containing simple carbohydrate is the source of the sugar. Milk, fruits, and vegetables contain naturally occurring sugars such as lactose and fructose. Refined carbohydrate typically contains white sugar, high fructose corn syrup (HFCS), or other highly processed sugars that do not occur naturally and are a concentrated source of calories. When sugars occur naturally in foods, they are usually in low concentrations and are just one of many nutrients that the food supplies. In contrast, when refined carbohydrate is added to foods or beverages, it is generally added in high concentrations. Because the carbohydrate is in concentrated form, these foods are relatively high in calories. The average adult in the United States consumes more than 300 kilocalories per day from the sugar added to food, which is too much for most people, especially if they are trying to lose weight.

Many people tend to think of complex carbohydrate as good, and they view simple carbohydrate, especially sugar, as bad, but the focus should be on when and how often you choose them. Much of the time you want to choose complex carbohydrate because it provides energy and a variety of other nutrients. Sometimes, however, the best choice will be a simple carbohydrate (for example, a beverage with sugar) because you need quick energy that you can easily absorb and digest, such as during or immediately after exercise. The choice is a balancing act, but generally the scales tip toward choosing complex carbohydrate much of the time.

Fiber

Fiber is a type of carbohydrate, but it is different from sugars and starches because it is not digested or absorbed from the intestinal tract. For that reason, fiber does not provide energy or calories, but it does help to regulate the digestive system and promote good health. Women should consume 25 grams of fiber each day and men 38 grams daily. The average fiber intake of both athletes and nonathletes in the United States is 15 to 19 grams daily.

Fiber is found in foods that contain complex carbohydrate (that is, whole grains, beans, tubers) and in fruits and vegetables, another reason that athletes should focus on those foods. Fruit and vegetable juices and refined carbohydrate are low in fiber, and sugars do not provide any fiber. When you consume too many foods with refined carbohydrate, your diet will likely be low in fiber, vitamins, and minerals.

Protein

Proteins are made up of amino acids, the building blocks for all protein. One of the primary roles of protein is to supply amino acids for building tissue, which is of particular interest to athletes because increasing muscle mass can improve training and performance. There are 20 different amino acids. Eight of these are considered essential, which in this sense means that the body cannot make these amino acids so they must be provided by protein-containing foods. The body manufactures the remaining 12 amino acids.

The amino acid content of the body is always in flux (known as protein balance) because muscle is both built and broken down in response to resistance training. Consuming protein-containing foods on a daily basis helps keep the body in protein balance. Look again at table 5.1 and note that protein provides energy, promotes growth and development, and regulates body functions. Protein is at the bottom of the energy column because protein should not be a primary source of energy. Instead, protein should be used to do what it does best—build tissue and help regulate body processes.

The protein intake for athletes in training is estimated at 1 to 2 grams per kilogram of body weight daily (or about 12 to 20 percent of total calories). As shown in table 5.5, this range covers a variety of needs, from those of recreational athletes who are beginning a training and conditioning program to the needs of well-conditioned strength athletes who are in a muscle-building phase. Athletes who are trying to lose body fat but maintain muscle mass often use the middle of this range, 1.5 grams per kilogram of body weight daily. Athletes who are trying to build muscle mass consume protein in amounts nearer the top end of the range.

TABLE 5.5

Estimated Daily Protein Need

Activity level or diet type	Daily protein needs (g/kg)
Recreational athlete not in training	1.0
Endurance athlete	1.2–1.4
Weight-loss diet (minimum needed)	1.5
Muscle-building diet	1.6–1.8
Ultraendurance athlete (rigorous training phase)	2.0

Fat

Fat is important because it provides energy when you are doing low- to moderate-intensity exercise, but certain fat found in food and the amount of excess body fat that you have can increase the risk for heart disease. Most fats are triglycerides, which are stored in muscle in small amounts and in adipose tissue (body fat) in large amounts. Some stored fat in the body allows athletes to perform low- to moderate-intensity exercise for long periods. Excessive storage fat, however, can impede performance and is detrimental to health.

The types of fatty acids that you consume make a difference to your health. Fats are either saturated, polyunsaturated, or monounsaturated. An excess intake of saturated fat increases the risk for heart disease because saturated fat influences the liver to make more of the carriers that deposit fat in arteries. When too much fat collects along the walls of the arteries, the arteries harden and blood flow to the heart is reduced, resulting in heart damage. Polyunsaturated and monounsaturated fats have been designated as heart-healthy fats because they lower the risk for heart disease.

As with simple and complex carbohydrate, choosing the types of fat to consume is a balancing act. Heart-healthy fat should be emphasized, and saturated fat should be limited. To accomplish a healthful balance, you need to be aware of the kinds of foods that contain each type of fat. Saturated fat is found in the greatest amounts in animal fats (for example, whole milk, cheese, fatty meats) and palm kernel and coconut oils, which are ingredients in many snack foods. Heart-healthy fat is found in vegetable oils, fish, nuts, and green leafy vegetables. Corn and safflower oils, fatty fish such as tuna and salmon, nuts and seeds, soybeans, and green leafy vegetables provide polyunsaturated fat. Olive and canola oil are examples of foods that have high amounts of monounsaturated fatty acids. By routinely choosing heart-healthy fat, you meet both your energy needs and your health needs.

Athletes in training should consume about 1 to 2 grams of fat per kilogram of body weight daily (or 20 to 30 percent of total calories). Fat intake should not typically dip below 1 gram per kilogram of body weight per day. The amount of fat that you need depends partly on your protein and carbohydrate needs, which you should determine first. Your fat needs also depend on whether you wish to gain weight primarily as muscle mass, lose weight primarily as body fat, or build muscle and lose body fat at the same time.

Vitamins and Minerals

Vitamins and minerals are known as micronutrients because they are needed in relatively small amounts to promote growth and development and to regulate body processes. Many of these processes, such as energy metabolism, red blood cell formation, and antioxidant functions, are important to optimal athletic training and performance.

Each of the following vitamins has more than one critical function:

Vitamin A	Vitamin B_1 (thiamin)	Vitamin C
Vitamin D	Vitamin B_2 (riboflavin)	Folate (folic acid)
Vitamin E	Vitamin B_3 (niacin)	Pantothenic acid
Vitamin K	Vitamin B_6	Biotin
	Vitamin B_{12}	

Athletes can meet the daily recommendations for all the vitamins from food alone if two conditions are met: adequate calorie intake and consumption of a variety of vitamin-rich foods. To ensure that they are getting enough vitamins, athletes should meet the Dietary Reference Intake (DRI) for vitamins (see table 5.6). These guidelines were developed for the lightly active general population, but they are applicable to most athletes because the DRI have a built-in margin of safety that should cover any increased need that is a result of exercise.

Numerous studies have shown that athletes often restrict their calorie intake and that in the process they restrict their intake of one or more vitamins. Turning to a one-a-day vitamin supplement would seem to be a logical and convenient way to supply the missing vitamins. The problem with this approach is that the athlete has only addressed one issue—the lack of certain vitamins—and not the underlying problems that usually occur with restricted caloric intake, which may include inadequate intake of carbohydrate, protein, fiber, and the minerals calcium and iron. The vitamin

TABLE 5.6

Dietary Reference Intakes (DRI) for Vitamins

Vitamin	AMOUNT PER DAY FOR MALES				AMOUNT PER DAY FOR NONPREGNANT FEMALES			
	14–18 years	19–30 years	31–50 years	51–70 years	14–18 years	19–30 years	31–50 years	51–70 years
A (mcg)	900	900	900	900	700	700	700	700
D (mcg)	5	5	5	10	5	5	5	10
E (mg)	15	15	15	15	15	15	15	15
K (mcg)	75	120	120	120	75	90	90	90
B_1 (thiamin) (mg)	1.2	1.2	1.2	1.2	1.0	1.1	1.1	1.1
B_2 (riboflavin) (mg)	1.3	1.3	1.3	1.3	1.0	1.1	1.1	1.1
B_3 (niacin) (mg)	16	16	16	16	14	14	14	14
B_6 (mg)	1.3	1.3	1.3	1.7	1.2	1.3	1.3	1.5
B_{12} (mcg)	2.4	2.4	2.4	2.4	2.4	2.4	2.4	2.4
C (mg)	75	90	90	90	65	75	75	75
Folate (folic acid) (mcg)	400	400	400	400	400	400	400	400
Pantothenic acid (mg)	5	5	5	5	5	5	5	5
Biotin (mcg)	25	30	30	30	25	30	30	30
Choline (mg)	550	550	550	550	400	425	425	425

For additional information about the DRI, see appendix A.

Reprinted, by permission, from the National Academies Press, Copyright 2005, National Academy of Sciences.

Source: *Dietary Reference Intakes for Energy, Carbohydrate, Fiber, Fat, Fatty Acids, Cholesterol, Protein, and Amino Acids (Macronutrients)*, pp. 1320-1321.

supplement approach is a bit like taking your car to a mechanic, learning that it has numerous problems, but choosing to fix just one of the problems. Eventually, the performance of your car will deteriorate.

But the problem with low vitamin intake is not caused only by low calorie intake. Some athletes take in sufficient calories, but because they do not eat nutritious foods, such as complex carbohydrate, fruits, and vegetables, they do not get enough vitamins, fiber, and other important nutrients. This result can easily occur when athletes eat or drink foods high in sugar, fat, and alcohol. These athletes are actually malnourished, not because they get too few calories but because they consume too few vitamins, minerals, fiber, and other important nutrients. Complete nutrition goes hand in hand with consuming the right amount of calories from a balance of carbohydrate-, protein-, and fat-containing foods in which vitamins occur naturally in the right proportions. Thus, athletes should focus on eating vitamin-containing foods rather than relying on a vitamin supplement.

Minerals found in relatively large amounts in the body include calcium, sodium, potassium, and chloride. These minerals are also electrolytes because they have either a positive or a negative charge. Electrolytes are essential for maintaining fluid balance (see chapter 8) and for proper heart, nerve, and muscle function. Trace minerals, such as iron and zinc, are found in relatively small amounts in the body.

The following minerals are essential because they promote growth and development and regulate body processes:

Calcium	Vanadium	Nickel
Phosphorus	Iron	Manganese
Sodium	Copper	Molybdenum
Potassium	Magnesium	Cobalt
Chloride	Zinc	Selenium
Sulfur	Fluoride	Silicon
Chromium	Iodine	Boron

From both an exercise and a health perspective all the minerals are important, but trying to deal with all 21 would quickly become overwhelming. Athletes often focus on just two—the calcium and iron found in food. This approach makes sense for many reasons. First, when the intake of calcium and iron from food is adequate, then the intake of the other 19 minerals is usually adequate. Second, iron is central to proper red blood cell formation, and low iron intake can eventually have a negative effect on training and performance. Third, low calcium and iron intake leads to specific diseases such as osteoporosis and iron-deficiency anemia.

Surveys show that many athletes are deficient in one or more minerals, often in both calcium and iron, because of poor food choices and lack of food intake. A low calorie intake limits the amount of minerals that a person might consume. Poor food choices are a particular problem with minerals because most foods do not have a large amount of any one mineral. For that reason minerals need to be obtained from a variety of nutritious foods. When athletes restrict their food intake or do not eat a variety of foods, they may be unable to obtain the total amount needed each day.

Athletes may think that calcium or iron supplementation would be a simple solution. Remember, however, that obtaining the proper amount of calcium and iron from foods increases the likelihood that you will consume the other 19 minerals that you need. A focus on calcium and iron supplements may solve the well-recognized problems, but it will not address other mineral deficiencies. A good philosophy to follow is to eat food first and supplement if necessary.

To ensure that you are getting enough minerals to support training, conditioning, and good health, you should meet the Dietary Reference Intake (DRI) for minerals (see table 5.7). As with the DRI for vitamins, these guide-

TABLE 5.7

Dietary Reference Intakes (DRI) for Minerals*

Mineral	AMOUNT PER DAY FOR MALES				AMOUNT PER DAY FOR NONPREGNANT FEMALES			
	14–18 years	19–30 years	31–50 years	51–70 years	14–18 years	19–30 years	31–50 years	51–70 years
Calcium (mg)	1,300	1,000	1,000	1,200	1,300	1,000	1,000	1,200
Phosphorus (mg)	1,250	700	700	700	1,250	700	700	700
Sodium (g)**	1.5	1.5	1.5	1.3	1.5	1.5	1.5	1.3
Potassium (g)	4.7	4.7	4.7	4.7	4.7	4.7	4.7	4.7
Chloride (g)	2.3	2.3	2.3	2.0	2.3	2.3	2.3	2.0
Chromium (mcg)	35	35	35	30	24	25	25	20
Iron (mg)	11	8	8	8	15	18	18	8
Copper (mcg)	890	900	900	900	890	900	900	900
Magnesium (mg)	410	400	420	420	360	310	320	320
Zinc (mg)	11	11	11	11	9	8	8	8
Fluoride (mg)	3	4	4	4	3	3	3	3
Iodine (mcg)	150	150	150	150	150	150	150	150
Manganese (mg)	2.2	2.3	2.3	2.3	1.6	1.8	1.8	1.8
Molybdenum (mcg)	43	45	45	45	43	45	45	45
Selenium (mcg)	55	55	55	55	55	55	55	55

* Boron, nickel, silicon, and vanadium are not included because a DRI has not been established. Excess levels are known to be toxic. Sulfur and cobalt are accounted for in protein and vitamin B_{12} recommendations, respectively. For additional information about the DRI, see appendix A.
**Values listed do not apply to athletes who lose substantial sodium in sweat.
Reprinted, by permission, from the National Academies Press, Copyright 2005, National Academy of Sciences.
Source: *Dietary Reference Intakes for Energy, Carbohydrate, Fiber, Fat, Fatty Acids, Cholesterol, Protein, and Amino Acids (Macronutrients)*, pp. 1322-1323.

lines were developed for the lightly active general population, but they are applicable to most athletes because the DRI have a built-in margin of safety. This margin of safety likely covers any increased need that is a result of exercise. One notable exception is sodium in athletes who lose a substantial amount in sweat. These athletes need to replenish the large amount of sodium that they lose daily, and the amount of sodium recommended by the DRI would fall short. Apart from this exception, the DRI for minerals is a good guideline for athletes to follow.

Water

Water is often listed last among the essential nutrients, but by rights it should be listed first because water is indispensable. If neither food nor water were available, you would die from lack of water, not from lack of food. Water helps regulate body temperature, transport nutrients and waste products, and is a vital part of every fluid in the body, such as blood. By weight, you need more water than you do any other nutrient. The relatively heavy weight of water is one reason that athletes who are trying to make weight manipulate the amount of water in the body. Water is so important that it gets its own chapter in this book—chapter 8.

Nutrition Selection and Timing

Just as nutrition and training go hand in hand, calories and nutrients go hand in hand. To meet your muscle-building and fat-loss goals, the key is choosing nutrient-dense foods, those foods rich in nutrients for the calories that they provide. In other words, nutrient-dense foods give you more bang (nutrients) for your buck (calories). Conversely, nutrient-poor foods are usually high in calories, typically from refined carbohydrate, fat, and alcohol, but they supply few essential nutrients. Consider these foods freeloaders because they take up calories but do not contribute enough nutrients to help the body do its work. Eating too many nutrient-poor foods can keep you from achieving your weight and body-composition goals and impede peak performance.

The timing of food intake across the day is important for proper training and performance and for changing weight and body composition. Athletes generally benefit from taking in some food or fluid before a training session. Some athletes also need food and fluid during training, and all athletes need food and fluid within the first hour after training. In other words, besides the total amount of calories, carbohydrate, protein, and fat that you need for one day, you also need to distribute them properly across the day. Distribution depends on when and how long you train on a given day.

The recovery period, a critical time for replenishment and rebuilding, begins immediately after exercise. During recovery, you must pay special

TABLE 5.8

Guidelines for Recovery Nutrition

Goal	Nutrients needed	Timing
Reestablish proper hydration	Water Sodium	Begin water intake immediately and continue drinking until all water lost during exercise has been replenished. If sodium losses are large, eat a salty snack immediately after exercise and then replenish sodium lost over the next 24 hours by lightly salting food.
Replenish muscle glycogen	Carbohydrate	Begin carbohydrate intake immediately and continue for the next 4 hours. Consume an adequate amount over the next 24 hours.
Resynthesize skeletal muscle tissue	Protein	Consume some protein as soon as possible (within the first hour) after exercise and an adequate amount of protein over the next 24 hours.
Resupply nutrients to counteract the stress of exercise	Vitamins Minerals	Consume an adequate amount (the DRI) of vitamins and minerals daily.

attention to the amount and timing of nutrient intake to make sure that your body is ready for the next training session. Table 5.8 outlines the goals during recovery and the nutrients needed to meet those goals. Note that some nutrients need to be consumed within the first hour after exercise, whereas others can be replenished over a longer period.

Athletes usually need to eat many times a day. A typical diet plan designed to support training, change body composition, and enhance performance includes three meals as well as snacks before and after exercise. This regimen is true for those who are trying to build muscle mass as well as for those who are trying to lose body fat, although the size of those meals and snacks will be different. But athletes face many constraints. One is time. Finding the time to shop, prepare, and eat meals or snacks may be difficult. Another is timing. Consuming foods at the right times is as important as consuming the right foods, so sometimes foods must be portable. Another critical issue is the form of the food—solid, semisolid, or liquid. A different form of food may be required to prevent gastrointestinal upset, which is common when food is consumed immediately before, during, and after high-intensity exercise.

You may find that you need to improve your cooking skills so that you can follow your diet plan and meet your body-composition goals. You may also want to use commercially prepared products that are essentially substitutes for foods. Among the most popular are meal replacement beverages; protein supplements in the form of powders, premade beverages, and bars; sport beverages; and carbohydrate gels. You can easily incorporate these products into your diet plan.

6

Adding Muscle, Gaining Mass

In chapter 4 you compared your personal measurements to successful athletes in your sport. This information formed the basis for setting your goals, one of which may be building muscle. Now you must answer some important questions: How much muscle should I build, and how can I do it? How long will it take me, and what do I need to know about timing? Increasing muscle mass requires an individually tailored program of resistance training coupled with a carefully designed nutrition strategy and dietary plan.

When it comes to building muscle, the ultimate goal is to add enough muscle mass to improve performance. The right amount of muscle mass, or lean mass, is based on the body composition that the athlete can safely and reasonably achieve and maintain and that best supports peak performance in a given sport and position. Although a greater percentage of lean mass is typically associated with greater power, that is not to say that the most effective goal is to gain as much muscle mass as possible. More is not always better. In some instances, too much muscle can be a hindrance. In fact, excess weight from muscle can damage joints and ligaments, reduce speed, and diminish agility.

Each athlete who wants to build muscle is likely to have a slightly different goal. For some, the goal is to gain only muscle because they do not need to gain or lose fat. But many athletes want to build muscle and change the amount of body fat as well. When current body weight is within an optimal range, increasing muscle mass may require the loss of some body fat. On the other hand, those who want to bulk up may want to gain muscle and increase body fat somewhat to reach a higher body weight and greater body mass.

Gaining muscle or gaining muscle and fat requires athletes to consume more calories than they expend. Doing that is relatively easy. By comparison, simultaneously adding muscle mass and losing body fat is much more difficult. Although the focus of this chapter is building muscle, do not lose sight of your other weight and body-composition goals.

Reasonable Expectations for Building Muscle

A male athlete who engages in a well-planned resistance-training program that is supported with an appropriate diet who does not use growth-enhancing drugs could reasonably expect to gain .5 to 1 pound (0.23 to 0.45 kilogram) of lean mass per week. A reasonable expectation for women is 50 to 75 percent of the gain for men, a weekly gain of 0.25 to 0.75 pound (0.11 to 0.34 kilogram). This weight gain includes an increase in the protein content of the muscle as well as an increase in muscle water and glycogen. Keep in mind that muscle building is a slow process.

Goals for increasing lean mass must factor in whether an athlete has been engaged in resistance training previously and, if so, how vigorously and for how long. Note that after the first year of resistance training, gains in lean mass will come less quickly. An untrained male who engages in a rigorous one-year resistance-training and nutrition program can increase body mass by approximately 20 percent, most of which will be lean mass. For example, a 180-pound (81.8-kilogram) untrained male could realistically expect to gain 36 pounds (16.4 kilograms) of weight with a rigorous one-year program. In subsequent years, however, the gain would slow considerably, typically to a 1 to 3 percent gain per year. At some point, additional gains may not be possible. A similar program for an untrained woman may result in about a 10 to 15 percent gain in body mass the first year and decreasing gains in subsequent years.

When to Build Muscle

The best time for most athletes to focus on increasing muscle mass is during the off-season and in the early preseason. During these periods athletes can do rigorous resistance training for muscle building (more weight or more repetitions) without overtraining or interfering with their usual training, conditioning, and skill development programs. During the later part of the preseason and during the competitive season, the focus changes to mainte-nance of muscle mass. Most athletes do not try to build muscle during the competitive season because doing so would likely interfere with training and undermine efforts to achieve peak performance in competition.

Athletes who would not adhere to this seasonal time frame include powerlifters and bodybuilders. Powerlifters who will easily qualify for their weight class typically try to continue to increase muscle mass up to the time of competition. Bodybuilders also increase muscle mass until they begin final preparations for a contest. In the final weeks before the contest, the focus changes to trying to maintain muscle while decreasing body fat to as low a level as possible.

How to Build Muscle

Three elements are required to build muscle mass: resistance exercise, calories, and protein. Resistance training and muscle growth require calories; therefore, a diet strategy that supports muscle building begins with ample calories, most of which should come from carbohydrate and fat. Furthermore, adequate energy intake in the form of carbohydrate and fat ensures that the body has enough fuel and does not catabolize, or break down, protein for energy instead of using it for muscle building. The primary purpose of protein is to supply amino acids, the required building blocks for creating muscle. Athletes may believe that they are consuming adequate or balanced diets until they examine their dietary intakes compared with their energy and nutrient needs.

Resistance Training

Resistance training, also known as weight training, uses the principle of overload to increase muscle mass. Through resistance exercise, you can place greater-than-normal stress on muscles by overloading them with greater-than-normal weight. In essence, you increase the volume of work that the muscles perform. Resistance training involves two components, weight and repetition, that combine to increase the volume of work and stress muscles. The stressed muscles respond to the overload of weight by growing in size and thus strengthening.

As your muscles grow stronger, you need to increase the workload to continue muscle growth. The demands of your sport and your performance goals will be important factors in determining the amount of weight and the number of repetitions you will use in your resistance-training program. Although a well-planned resistance-training program is critical, it is beyond the scope of this book. Refer to appendix A for more information about resistance training.

For overloaded muscles to grow, they must have readily available energy to perform the extra work plus the raw materials to build additional muscle. Thus, for maximum muscle gains, you should coordinate your weight-training regimen with a nutrition strategy and meal plan. In particular, you must consume the right amount of calories and the proper amounts and proportions of protein, carbohydrate, and fat. Precise training and nutrition create the best results. You would not train without a plan; therefore, you should not eat without one either.

Calories

If you begin a resistance-training program or increase the level of your current resistance-training program, you will need more calories because you are exercising more. Your body also needs additional calories to promote growth of muscle tissue. Therefore, you must determine how many calories you need while you are in a muscle-building phase. To do this, you first need a baseline estimate of how many calories you currently consume. The dietary analysis discussed in chapter 3 will give you this information.

Athletes who are eating adequate calories to maintain their baseline weight need to increase their calorie intake to gain body mass. Males should add approximately 400 to 500 kilocalories per day, and females should add approximately 300 to 400 kilocalories daily. Those who want to gain some body fat in addition to the gain in muscle should choose the higher end of this range. For example, a 161-pound (73-kilogram) male who is currently moderately active has baseline caloric needs of about 3,000 kilocalories daily. If he begins a rigorous resistance-training program to increase muscle mass, he should increase his caloric intake to approximately 3,400 to 3,500 kilocalories daily.

If you wish to increase muscle mass and decrease body fat simultaneously, you must be more precise with your caloric estimate. As a starting point, you must closely estimate your baseline calories. Increasing muscle mass is a growth state, which requires you to consume more calories than your baseline intake. Decreasing body fat requires a calorie deficit, which usually involves taking in fewer calories than your baseline intake. To achieve both goals at the same time, some of the calories needed for growth must come from stored fat. For simultaneous muscle gain and fat loss, females should increase baseline intake by about 200 kilocalories daily and males should add about 300 kilocalories each day.

These guidelines are a good starting point, but you will need to fine-tune them to determine the proper amount of calories for you each day. If you take in too many calories you will gain too much body fat, but if you take in too few calories you will not be able to build muscle. Determining the correct intake of calories is not easy because when you start a muscle-building program, you must consider two factors that influence caloric intake: the number of calories that you expend in resistance training and the effect that an increase in muscle mass has on resting metabolic rate (RMR).

Caloric expenditure during a rigorous resistance-training program is approximately 10 kilocalories per minute for men and 7 kilocalories per minute for women. In other words, one hour of rigorous resistance training burns about 600 kilocalories in men and 420 kilocalories in women. This level of calorie expenditure is for the actual time spent lifting weights, which does not include the time spent resting between sets. For example, an untrained female who begins a resistance-training program may lift for a total of 30 minutes, resulting in a calorie expenditure of about 200 kilocalories. Accounting for this additional energy expenditure is one of the reasons that females who want to build muscle mass are advised to consume an additional 300 to 400 kilocalories daily.

You must also take into account the effect of an increase in lean body mass on your resting metabolic rate. Research suggests that a cumulative training effect of sustained, regular exercise may slightly raise RMR. Increasing the total amount of muscle mass also increases RMR. These increases in RMR raise your baseline caloric needs. Therefore, as you add resistance training and increase muscle mass, you will need more calories than you did before. As explained in chapter 3, physical activity and resting metabolic rate are the two major factors that affect your total energy expenditure.

RMR typically has the most influence on total energy expenditure (TEE). As your percentage of lean mass increases, RMR increases; a lower percentage of lean mass would result in a lower RMR. Increasing lean mass is one of the most effective ways to increase RMR. But other relationships are important as well. For instance, daily caloric intake is very important. As shown in figure 6.1, an appropriate energy intake in combination with resistance exercise can significantly increase total lean mass, which increases RMR. Consuming sufficient calories also has a direct effect on RMR, although the increase is small.

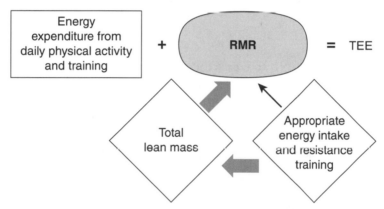

Figure 6.1　Appropriate energy intake in combination with resistance exercise can increase total lean mass, which in turn increases RMR. RMR is a major influence on TEE.
RMR = resting metabolic rate; TEE = total energy expenditure.

In contrast, severely restricting calories for a length of time can suppress RMR, as shown in figure 6.2. Without appropriate calorie intake, an athlete cannot build muscle so total lean mass cannot increase. Furthermore, RMR will be suppressed because the athlete is in a state of semistarvation when calories are severely restricted over time (see the Physiology of Weight Loss section in chapter 7). The suppressed RMR limits an athlete's ability to perform work or physical activity, which reduces energy expenditure and may negatively affect performance.

An often overlooked but important consideration when determining a recommended calorie range is a comparison of an athlete's usual energy intake with predicted energy requirement. Athletes may believe that they are consuming adequate or balanced diets until they examine their dietary intake compared with their energy and nutrient needs. Proper caloric intake is critical to muscle growth. To consume enough calories to build muscle, you need to eat both meals and snacks. Many athletes find that they need to eat three meals and two or three snacks each day. The snacks are part of the daily total energy intake.

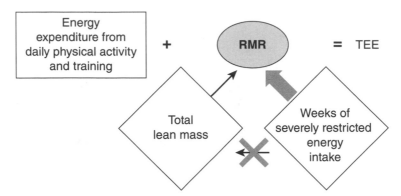

Figure 6.2 Prolonged restricted energy intake prevents an increase in total lean mass and decreases RMR.
RMR = resting metabolic rate; TEE = total energy expenditure.

Carbohydrate. Carbohydrate is the primary fuel for exercising muscles and is essential for muscle building. It is also the preferred fuel for the brain and nervous system. The body uses and depletes more carbohydrate during high-intensity exercise than it does protein or fat. Dietary carbohydrate restores muscle glycogen stores depleted by high-intensity exercise such as rigorous resistance training, spares protein from being burned as energy so that it can be used to build muscle, and enhances tolerance to increased training, resulting in maintenance of performance, mood, and concentration. Without adequate intake of carbohydrate you will not have sufficient fuel to perform resistance exercise and build muscle. Carbohydrate from grain products, beans and legumes, vegetables, fruit, and milk should supply the greatest percentage of calories (energy) in a muscle-building diet. The proper amount of carbohydrate in a muscle-building diet is typically 7 to 8 grams per kilogram of body weight daily. Do not make the mistake of consuming too little carbohydrate.

Fat. Muscle building requires lots of calories. Many of the calories needed to support muscle growth come from carbohydrate, but fat is an important source as well. Some athletes who are trying to gain muscle mass need to focus on getting sufficient dietary fat so that they can consume enough calories daily. Dietary fat is necessary to replenish intramuscular fat stores, manufacture hormones, and absorb fat-soluble vitamins. Essential fatty acids must come from dietary sources found in foods such as leafy green vegetables, vegetable oils, nuts and seeds, and fatty fish. Not all dietary sources of fat, however, are equally healthful. High intakes of some forms of dietary fats can be detrimental to health. For good health and optimal performance, most fat should be from fish or from plant sources, such as oils, nuts, and seeds. The amount of fat that athletes need daily depends on the amount of protein and carbohydrate needed. Fat will fill in the remaining calories.

Protein

Protein supplies the raw material for muscle building by furnishing the body with amino acids, which are the structural components of muscle. To build lean mass effectively, you need to be in positive protein balance so that your body has the building material needed to create new muscle tissue. To maintain positive protein balance, calorie intake must be sufficient to allow protein to be used for tissue building rather than for energy. Most highly trained athletes' energy needs are high, and rigorous resistance training adds an additional energy demand, so to build muscle, you must consume enough calories as well as a sufficient amount of protein.

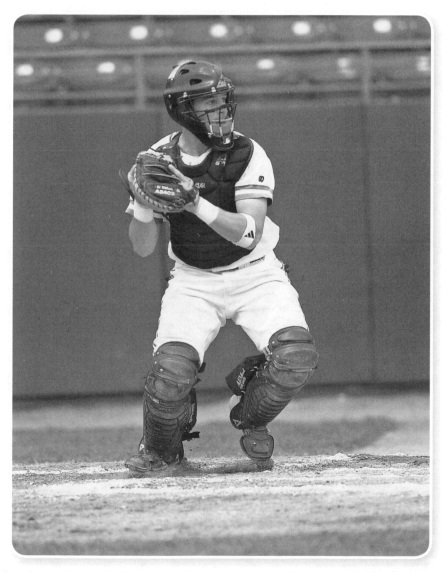

Catchers frequently need to build muscle for explosive power. To accomplish this goal, they must consume adequate calories and enough protein to maintain a positive protein balance.

For those intending to build muscle mass through a resistance-training program, the recommendation for protein intake is typically 1.6 to 1.8 grams per kilogram of body weight daily. This guideline is based on the assumption that calorie intake is adequate. Strength athletes often consume between 1.5 to 2.0 grams per kilogram of body weight daily, so meeting this recommendation is not difficult.

Some athletes mistakenly believe that extra protein will help them train harder and gain muscle faster. Research has demonstrated that daily protein intake beyond 2 grams per kilogram of body weight does not enhance work capacity or performance. Excess protein does not cause muscle to grow faster. Protein intake exceeding 2 grams per kilogram per day is burned for energy or converted to fat and stored in adipose tissue rather than being used for additional muscle building. Despite strongly held beliefs of some coaches, trainers, and athletes, no benefits result from excessive protein intake and, in fact, it can cause the following problems:

■ **Lowered carbohydrate intake**. Excessive protein intake throws off the balance of calories from carbohydrate, protein, and fat by providing calories that should be supplied by carbohydrate. Low carbohydrate intake reduces the ability to restore muscle glycogen after training and hinders the ability to train maximally.

■ **Excessive caloric intake**. If protein intake is excessive and no adjustment is made in total calorie intake, excessive protein will add extra calories, resulting in an unwanted gain in body fat.

■ **Greater fluid losses**. Excessive protein intake increases the need for water to flush the waste products of protein metabolism out of the body through the kidneys.

■ **Higher food costs**. An overlooked consequence of excessive protein is the unnecessary cost, because protein foods are often more expensive than carbohydrate foods such as grains, beans, and legumes. Some protein supplements are more expensive than protein foods and are no more effective than high-quality food protein in helping to build muscle.

Timing Protein and Carbohydrate Intake

A growing body of research suggests that just before resistance training and immediately afterward are key times for athletes to consume a protein and carbohydrate snack to support optimal muscle building. Resistance training stimulates protein synthesis, but the training also breaks down muscle protein and creates a temporary negative protein balance. Eventually, protein synthesis will be greater than protein breakdown, but proper nutrition is needed for this to occur. As part of an overall nutrition plan, protein and carbohydrate intake before and after resistance exercise helps maximize protein synthesis and minimize protein breakdown and negative balance. To gain full benefit from your pre- and postexercise snacks, be sure to include ample fluids.

Preexercise Snack

A protein and carbohydrate snack before resistance training can help to maximize the training session, although more research is needed on this topic. The carbohydrate provides needed calories and helps maintain blood glucose. A small amount of protein (about 6 to 10 grams) with carbohydrate may help reduce muscle protein breakdown and supply additional amino acids. As an example, one pack (two bars) of whole-grain oats and nut granola bars and 24 ounces (720 milliliters) of a sports beverage (such as Gatorade, Powerade, Accelerade, All Sport) would provide approximately 6 to 8 grams of protein and 60 grams of carbohydrate. These foods would be an appropriate preexercise snack for a 100-kilogram (220-pound) athlete. The snack should be consumed one hour before exercise.

Postexercise Snack

Resistance training breaks down muscle protein, and the hour immediately following training is an opportune time to repair and build muscle. Take full advantage and consume a postexercise snack that contains both high quality protein and carbohydrate. Studies show that consuming at least 6 to 12 grams of essential amino acids (the equivalent of 10 to 20 grams of high-quality protein) immediately after resistance exercise promotes muscle growth by enhancing muscle protein balance and increasing muscle protein synthesis. Research also shows that muscle protein balance improves when 1 gram of carbohydrate per kilogram of body weight is consumed immediately after exercise. For example, an athlete who weighs 220 pounds (100 kilograms) should consume at least 10 grams of protein and 100 grams of carbohydrate after resistance training to maximize muscle gains.

Protein of high biological value (for example, milk and other animal protein) provides the essential amino acids needed to optimize muscle growth. For example, 8 ounces (240 grams) of fat-free yogurt provides about 10 to 14 grams of protein (6 grams of essential amino acids). Protein supplements can be used effectively to facilitate the ideal timing of protein consumption, but as with food, they must be calculated as part of your overall nutrition intake. Some protein supplements may be more convenient to carry with you if they do not need refrigeration, but they may be expensive or not appeal to your taste. Choose the protein source that works best for you. Milk, yogurt, grains such as granola or energy bars, fruits, and sports beverages provide carbohydrate. Table 6.1 lists the protein and carbohydrate content of some postexercise snacks.

TABLE 6.1

Protein and Carbohydrate Content of Selected Snacks

Snack	Protein (g)	Carbohydrate (g)
8 oz (240 ml) low-fat cow's or soy milk	8	12
6 oz (180 g) low-fat fruit yogurt	6	25
8 oz (240 ml) low-fat kefir	14	25
12 oz (360 ml) low-fat chocolate milk	12	42
8 oz (240 ml) high-protein recovery drink	14	30
2 cups (80 g) whole-grain cereal with 8 oz (240 ml) nonfat milk	14	56
2 large eggs on 2 slices of whole-wheat toast	20	28
3 oz (90 g) turkey breast on 2 slices of whole-wheat bread	32	24
3 tbsp (48 g) peanut butter and 2 tbsp (42 g) honey on 3 slices of whole-wheat bread	20	82

Planning for Optimal Body Weight and Composition

Although the focus of this chapter so far has been on muscle building, you may want to gain or lose body fat at the same time. Take the case of Morgan, a 6-foot, 157-pound (183-centimeter, 71.4-kilogram) 17-year-old high school male baseball outfielder who aspired to earn a college baseball scholarship. A body-composition assessment estimated Morgan's body fat at 9.4 percent and lean mass at 90.6 percent (see table 6.2). At his baseline weight of 157 pounds (71.4 kilograms) he has 142 pounds (64.5 kilograms) of lean mass and 15 pounds (6.8 kilograms) of body fat. Surveys of Division I collegiate outfielders reported an average body fat of 11 percent. The players at the school he wanted to attend weighed an average of 170 to 190 pounds (77.3 to 86.4 kilograms)

TABLE 6.2

Body-Composition Goals for a High School Baseball Player

Physical assessments	College baseball outfielders	Morgan's baseline measurements	Morgan's goals
Height		6 ft (183 cm)	
Weight		157 lb (71.4 kg)	187 lb (85 kg)
Body composition Body fat Lean mass	11% 89%	9.4% (15 lb or 6.8 kg) 90.6% (142 lb or 64.5 kg)	13% (25 lb or 11.4 kg) 87% (162 lb or 73.6 kg)

One of Morgan's goals was to gain weight by adding lean mass to increase power, strength, and sprint speed before his senior year baseball season, eight months away. Another goal was to gain some body fat to add some size and be more comparable to a college player. Morgan began a rigorous resistance-training program. He could realistically expect to achieve up to a 20 percent increase in total body mass over a year. Besides stepping up his training, Morgan increased his caloric intake by 500 kilocalories daily by adding two substantial snacks to the meals that his mother prepared for him. He ate a turkey sandwich as an after-school snack and a large bowl of cereal with milk as an after-dinner snack. By graduation, Morgan had gained 30 pounds (13.6 kilograms), which consisted of about 20 pounds (9 kilograms) of muscle mass and about 10 pounds (4.5 kilograms) of body fat.

Now consider the case of Scott. He is a 6-foot 1-inch, 237-pound (185-centimeter, 107.7-kilogram) water polo player with body fat of 18 percent (43 pounds, or 19.5 kilograms) and 194 pounds (88.2 kilograms) of lean mass (see table 6.3). He wanted to be "ripped" by training camp. He was working to become the strongest and quickest swimmer on the team and earn a starting position. To do this, he needed to gain strength and increase speed and agility. He decided that during the remaining four weeks of conditioning before training camp he would cut his total weight to 222 pounds (101 kilograms), trim his body fat to 9 percent to increase speed and agility, and gain strength by increasing lean mass by 8 pounds (3.6 kilograms). A 15-pound (6.8-kilogram) total weight loss that included an 8-pound (3.6-kilogram) gain in lean body mass sounded realistic to Scott, but was it?

Scott began to restrict his food intake so that he would lose body fat. He added rigorous resistance training to his usual water polo training but found that he was feeling more fatigued than in the past. He was not keeping up with his teammates in the gym or increasing his muscle size, so he decided to follow a high-protein, low-carbohydrate diet. At the end of the four-week conditioning period he had not lost any body fat or added any muscle mass.

TABLE 6.3

Body-Composition Goals for a Water Polo Player

Physical assessments	Scott's baseline measurements	Scott's unrealistic goals	Realistic goals for Scott
Height	6 ft 1 in. (185 cm)		
Weight	237 lb (107.7 kg)	222 lb (101 kg)	230 lbs (104.5 kg)
Body composition Body fat Lean mass	18.0% (43 lb or 19.5 kg) 82.0% (194 lb or 88.2 kg)	9.0% (20 lb or 9 kg) 91.0% (202 lb or 91.8 kg)	15% (34.5 lb or 15.7 kg) 85% (195.5 lb or 88.9 kg)

This example illustrates a common scenario for many athletes. First, Scott set unrealistic goals. Second, he used a strategy that did not take into account that muscle growth requires caloric and nutritional support. Scott wanted to gain substantial muscle mass while shedding body fat, and he sought to do both in a short time. His goals, 222 pounds (101 kilograms) and 9 percent body fat, required a 23-pound (10.5-kilogram) loss of body fat. Even under the best conditions (rigorous resistance training, an equally vigorous cardiovascular exercise plan, and a carefully planned dietary intake), it would be difficult, if not impossible, to build muscle mass and lose 4 pounds (1.8 kilograms) per week for four weeks. Scott did not start the process early enough to achieve his goals. Changing weight and body composition takes time, and planning is essential. A more realistic goal would be to aim for a 1- to 2-pound (0.45- to 0.9-kilogram) loss of fat per week and a 0.5-pound (.23-kilogram) gain of lean mass per week. With a carefully balanced nutrition and exercise regimen and a controlled calorie intake, a reasonable expectation over four weeks would be a weight range of 228 to 231 pounds (103.6 to 105 kilograms), 15 to 16 percent body fat, and a 2- to 4-pound (0.9- to 1.8-kilogram) gain in lean body mass. Given the time that he had available, his goal of a loss of 23 pounds (10.5 kilograms) of fat and a gain of 8 pounds (3.6 kilograms) of lean mass was not realistic. A practical goal would have been a 1.5-pound (0.7-kilogram) increase in lean mass and up to an 8.5-pound (3.8-kilogram) loss of fat.

Trying to increase muscle mass and lose body fat at the same time is not easy because you are essentially asking the body to go in opposite directions. You may find it better to focus on building muscle mass first, which may also result in a small increase in body fat, and then fine-tune your body composition by losing any unwanted body fat. Either way you must have a plan that allows you enough time to reach your goals.

Realistic expectations are critical to effective muscle building. With a well-designed plan, a potential gain of .5 to 1 pound (0.23 to 0.45 kilogram) per week can be used to establish your time frame. If your goal is to add 10 pounds (4.5 kilograms) of muscle, you will need from 10 to 20 weeks to reach that goal. As you chart your course for success, be sure to address four essential components of a muscle-building diet to maximize the effects of your resistance training:

- Ample calories (energy)
- The right balance of carbohydrate, protein, and fat
- Nutrient density (maximum amount of nutrients for the calories provided)
- Proper timing of your meals and snacks for maximum recovery

Remember that even with a carefully planned strategy, your weight gain will likely include some body fat. By precisely planning your diet, you can minimize fat gain while maximizing muscle gain.

Evaluation and Reassessment

Increasing muscle mass takes time. Evaluating the results may not be realistic until you have followed your diet and resistance-training program for about a month. The best way to assess whether you are gaining muscle (and possibly losing body fat at the same time) is to remeasure your body composition every four to six weeks. Despite the fact that body weight does not tell the whole story, weekly weigh-ins do provide some indication of change. You can also take girth measurements and remeasure them monthly. If you also measured your metabolic rate, then a remeasurement would be beneficial, but changes in metabolic rate because of increases in muscle mass may not be evident for the first 10 weeks. Reassessments give you information to judge whether your diet plan and resistance-training program are working. The more objective information you have, the more precise the evaluation of your progress will be.

Evaluation is the foundation for making adjustments that keep you on course. Remember the adage "If you don't measure it, you can't manage it." If you have moved off course, you want to catch the blip early and make the necessary modifications to get back on track. The sooner you adjust, the better the chances are that you will reach your goal. For instance, if you are not gaining weight steadily and at the rate you have planned, perhaps you need more calories or a better-balanced calorie distribution that you can achieve by tweaking your pre- and postexercise snacks. If you are gaining weight but the weight is more fat weight than muscle, your calorie intake may be too great and you may need to trim it back slightly. Fatigue is a clue that your diet may not be supplying adequate energy, carbohydrate, nutrients, or fluids.

The best way to evaluate your progress is to post a chart (Track Your Progress in appendix B) with your goals and the measurements that you can make. As part of your plan, schedule your measurements at reasonable intervals and be ready to make modifications as needed.

Losing Fat, Winning Results

"I need to drop weight without losing strength, power, or endurance. How do I do this?" This is a common question from athletes. Even after performing a dedicated strength-training program and adding muscle mass, you may have more work to do. Your body may need to be lean, strong, *and* efficient. In many cases, improving efficiency means losing excess body fat because excess body weight hampers efficiency when you need to move your body.

Running, cycling, swimming, "ball" sports (basketball, soccer, tennis, lacrosse, hockey), field activities (high jumping), and acrobatic sports (figure skating, gymnastics) are just some examples of sports in which athletes benefit from not having excess body fat. Athletes in sports with weight classes, such as wrestlers, boxers, and martial artists, may also need to lose body fat to compete in a certain weight class. Athletes who choose to change their weight should think beyond the number on the scale. They must be concerned about effective weight loss because if losing weight means losing strength, then weight loss does not offer a performance advantage.

Weight Loss and Performance

Effective weight loss, not just weight loss, is needed to improve performance. Dropping weight does not make sense if the weight is mostly muscle and water. The key to effective weight loss is to lose excess body fat. Losing muscle mass, which happens when you restrict calories too much, is not effective because your power and performance can decline. Losing too much water weight is not effective or safe because dehydration affects performance and can lead to heat illness.

Many athletes, especially those beginning an intense training program, find that an initial loss of body fat is beneficial to performance. Well-trained athletes may also find that fine-tuning body composition by losing excess body fat has a positive influence on performance. But at some point additional loss of body fat is not advantageous. Furthermore, trying to reach an ever-lower percentage of body fat will eventually be harmful. In the quest to lose weight but not strength, power, or endurance, keep in mind that the end goal is peak performance, not a certain body weight.

Recreational distance runners, especially those who have not been lifelong runners, usually find that losing the extra fat around the waist helps improve performance. A 220-pound (100-kilogram) runner who loses 30 pounds (13.6 kilograms) of excess body fat is likely to be a more efficient runner at 190 pounds (86.4 kilograms). This is an example of effective weight loss for improved performance. But the elite female distance runner who is already lean and has virtually no excess body fat is unlikely to improve performance with further weight loss because the loss of weight is apt to be from muscle, water, or depleted glycogen stores. Under these circumstances, a decline in performance is likely. This is an example of ineffective weight loss because of the negative effect on performance.

Figures 7.1 and 7.2 illustrate the approaches and outcomes for a recreational and an elite runner. Both did assessments of height, weight, and body composition. Each stated a goal, although the elite runner's goal was

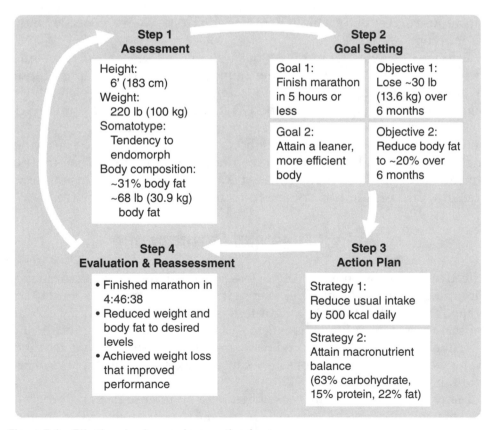

Figure 7.1   Effective plan for a male recreational runner.

less specific. The recreational runner set realistic objectives based on weight and body-composition assessment and devised a specific strategy to achieve those objectives within a reasonable time frame. In contrast, the elite runner had one (ill-conceived) objective, lower body weight, and did not consider which body components she would lose if she met this goal. Her action plan was not specific, and she focused only on restricting calories and fat. She achieved her objective (weight loss) but, sadly, not her goal (peak performance) because the weight loss impaired her performance.

Ineffective weight loss can result from the methods used to achieve it. Wrestlers and boxers have been known to use drastic measures over a short period to make weight. Starvation-type diets, excessive exercise in sauna suits, and use of diuretics and diet aids are examples of methods used to induce rapid weight loss. Often these athletes meet the first part of their goal, dropping weight, but fail to meet the second part of their goal, maintaining strength or power. Two key factors in effective weight loss are time and safety. The end goal is peak performance from loss of excess body fat, but to accomplish this goal the athlete must consider the time needed to achieve it safely.

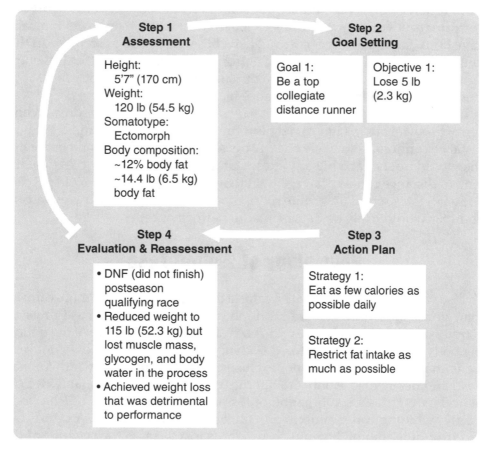

Figure 7.2   Ill-conceived plan for a female elite runner.

You should seek to maintain your level of training and performance while you are trying to lose body fat. Therefore, you should attempt to reach your weight-loss goal during the off-season and early in the preseason. Because the body has a greater need for energy and carbohydrate during competition or heavy training periods, restricting calories is more likely to be detrimental to performance at that time than it is at other times of the year. Nevertheless, weight loss may be a goal for the athlete at any time, and some athletes whose weight must be certified may need to lose weight up to the time of the weigh-in. The best approach is to plan so that you are not caught trying to reduce scale weight drastically in a short time. For example, large losses of weight may not be realistic during preseason training and conditioning camp, whereas small losses would be appropriate. Drastic measures are likely to have a negative effect on training, performance, and health.

Percent Body Fat and Performance

If aspiring athletes know the percentage body fat of the top athlete in their sport, they may think that they should achieve that same percentage. This assumption is erroneous because a specific percent body fat does not predict performance. For example, professional male ice hockey players typically have body fat in the range of 8 to 12 percent. Achieving a percentage in this range, however, does not mean that performance will improve. Such average figures may be a good guideline to pursue, but the percent body fat associated with *your* optimum performance may be outside this range.

Here is another way to look at it. If achieving an extremely low percentage of body fat always improved performance, then every champion female distance runner would likely have 12 percent body fat because, theoretically, she would not be carrying any excess fat. In fact, studies of successful elite female distance runners have shown that they range from 12 to 18 percent body fat. For some of these elite runners, striving to achieve a lower percent body fat would likely be detrimental to performance.

Physiology of Weight Loss

To lose weight, you must create a calorie deficit by expending more calories than you consume. To create a calorie deficit, you can increase physical activity or reduce food intake or do both. To make up for some of the deficit, the body releases fat from stored body fat. What most people do not realize is that the weight lost is not exclusively made up of body fat. We may wish and desire to lose only fat, but the body does not work that way. Loss of body weight is a combination of loss of body fat and loss of lean body mass, including water, muscle protein, and stored glycogen. A significant factor in determining how much weight is lost as fat is the severity of the calorie restriction.

Fasting and starvation-type diets are often popular with those whose goal is rapid weight loss. A drastic reduction in food intake might seem to be the fastest way to reduce body fat stores, but because the body's response to a severe lack of food is hormonally controlled, there are unintended, negative consequences of severe food restriction. The difference between fasting and starvation is only a matter of intent. The consequences are the same.

Studies have shown that when calorie restriction is severe, the loss of lean body mass is large. Even when a person tries to compensate for a severely restricted energy intake with a high-protein diet and resistance training, losses to lean body mass occur because the calorie deficit still plunges the body into a state of semistarvation. Diets that severely restrict calories are counterproductive for athletes because too much muscle, water, and glycogen are also lost. Remember that the goal is not just weight loss; the goal is improved performance, which results from effective weight loss.

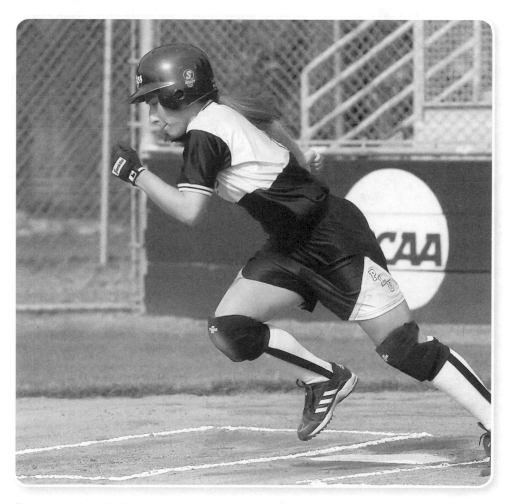

To gain speed, softball players often want to decrease body fat, but if they incur too large a calorie deficit they will lose lean body mass as well.

Think about weight loss from the body's perspective; it can die from starvation. Starvation is the result of prolonged fasting, which is abstaining from or severely limiting food for a long period. When the body is starved of sufficient energy, it goes into survival mode. To prevent starvation, the body makes small metabolic modifications when food is in short supply.

You may not connect a one- or two-day fast with starvation, but your body does. Fasting, even in the short term, forces the body to adjust to a lack of food, such as by reducing liver and muscle glycogen (the stored form of carbohydrate). In fact, liver glycogen stores are typically depleted within 12 to 18 hours after a fast, so the risk for a low blood sugar level and a negative effect on training and performance quickly materializes.

If a severe restriction of food intake continues, the body makes adjustments that are more substantial because it is moving toward starvation. One adjustment is to release fat from adipose tissue (a desirable consequence), but other adjustments include the breakdown of muscle protein to provide glucose and the use of fatty acids by muscle as a primary fuel. Remember that the preferred muscle fuel for high-intensity exercise is carbohydrate. Some of these adjustments are not desirable or beneficial, but they will occur if calories are severely restricted for more than two days.

A starvation-type diet also lowers the metabolic rate within just a few days because the body is trying to prevent substantial reduction of both lean and fat tissue. This consequence may seem illogical to the person who is trying to lose large amounts of body fat, but the body is trying to survive by protecting against the loss of any of its tissues. Think of this response as a body brownout, an efficient way to conserve energy. For example, the metabolic rate of a baseball player may fall from 1,550 to 1,390 kilocalories per day after two weeks when total food intake is limited to 1,200 kilocalories daily.

Moreover, not only does the body lower its metabolic rate while calories are being severely restricted, it maintains this lower rate after the starvation-type diet ends. The lower metabolic rate persists for weeks, not just a couple of days. When the baseball player increases his caloric intake, his metabolic rate will likely remain at about 1,400 kilocalories daily for a couple of weeks. For this reason, very low-calorie diets and severe caloric restriction often result in eventual weight gain and thus are not helpful to athletes.

So, if you want to lose weight, how do you signal your body that you do not intend to starve yourself? The best way is to avoid severely restricting caloric intake. A weight-reduction diet should involve a modest restriction of calories, but the degree of restriction is important. Each person is different, so there is no way to quantify what constitutes severe caloric restriction. In general, however, a person who loses more than 2 pounds (0.9 kilogram) of scale weight per week may be experiencing a severely restricted caloric intake.

A realistic expectation for athletes is to lose 1 to 2 pounds (0.45 to 0.9 kilogram) per week. Such a loss of scale weight will include some losses of muscle and water, especially in the early weeks, but most of the loss will be body fat. This recommendation takes into account that athletes still need to train and therefore should reduce calories only moderately. At the same time, athletes must not deprive themselves of a balanced intake of important nutrients such as protein, carbohydrate, and fat. If you follow a weight-loss diet that promises a 5- or 10-pound (2.3- to 4.5-kilogram) weight loss in a week, you will likely be unable to maintain training, performance, or proper hydration.

Strategies for Losing Fat

Obviously, severe calorie restriction is not recommended because too much lean body mass is lost and the metabolic rate is likely to fall. So, what is the best way to lose body fat and protect against unwanted physiological changes? Four basic factors work together: (1) moderate calorie restriction daily, (2) a diet that includes sufficient protein (but is still calorie restricted), (3) balanced intake of carbohydrate and fat, and (4) resistance exercise. This combination of factors is the best way for an athlete to lose body fat and protect against the loss of lean body mass, although some lean body mass is likely to be lost even under the best of circumstances.

Moderate Calorie Restriction

Adult athletes should consume a minimum of 30 kilocalories per kilogram of body weight daily. An athlete who weighs 60 kilograms (132 pounds) should not take in fewer than 1,800 kilocalories daily, and an athlete who weighs 50 kilograms (110 pounds) should not take in fewer than 1,500 kilocalories daily. At least 30 kilocalories per kilogram are needed to allow sufficient intake of protein to minimize loss of lean body mass and sufficient carbohydrate to restore some of the muscle glycogen used during training. Diets that provide fewer than 30 kilocalories per kilogram are also low in fat and are hard to follow over the weeks or months needed to meet weight-loss goals.

The guidelines in table 7.1 can help you avoid severe calorie restriction. If your weight falls between those given in the chart, then your minimum calorie level falls between the corresponding values. Note that your training

TABLE 7.1

Avoiding Severe Calorie Restriction

Weight (kg and lb)		Minimum calorie intake*
86.5 kg or more	190 lb or more	2,600 kcal daily
73 kg	160.5 lb	2,200 kcal daily
66.5 kg	146 lb	2,000 kcal daily
60 kg	132 lb	1,800 kcal daily
50 kg or less	110 lb or less	1,500 kcal daily

*These minimum calorie guidelines are for athletes who are trying to lose weight quickly but trying to avoid severe caloric restriction. If you experience exceptional fatigue or are unable to train or perform as usual, then the minimum is too low for you.

and conditioning program may be so rigorous that the minimum calorie level suggested in these guidelines may not be sufficient for you. Failing to take in sufficient calories could negatively affect your ability to train and perform.

Figures 7.3 and 7.4 illustrate some of the changes that can occur with calorie restriction depending on the amount of calories consumed daily. The first wrestler in figure 7.3 is well on his way to meeting his goals and objectives, but the wrestler in figure 7.4 undermined his efforts by choosing a weight-loss diet that was too low in calories.

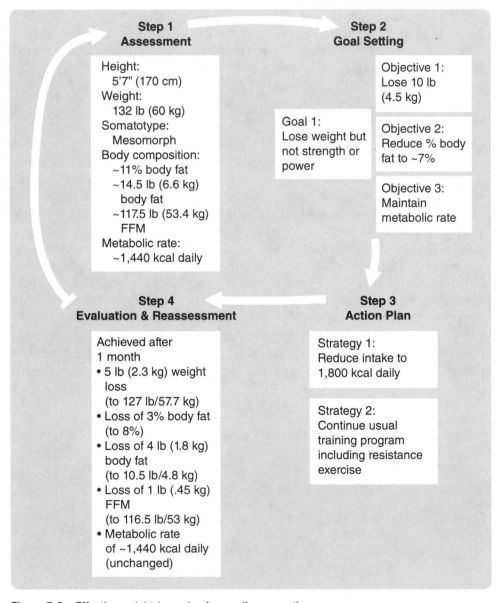

Figure 7.3 Effective weight-loss plan for a college wrestler.
FFM = fat-free mass (weight of muscle, bone, fluids, and organs).

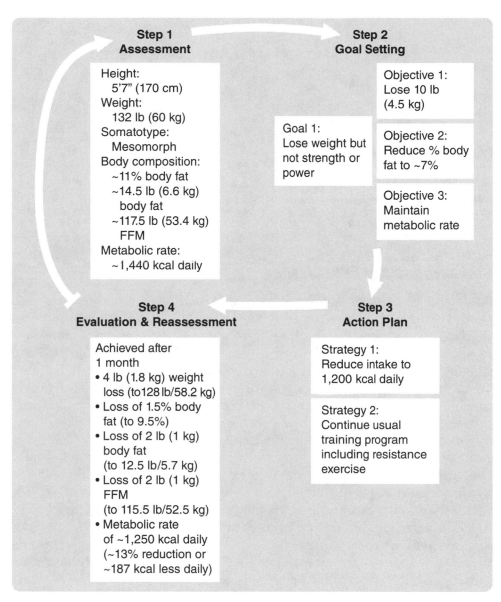

Figure 7.4 Ineffective weight-loss plan for a college wrestler.
FFM = fat-free mass (weight of muscle, bone, fluids, and organs).

Adequate Protein Intake

When athletes restrict calories to lose weight they need to make sure that they are getting enough protein. A daily protein intake of about 1.5 grams of protein per kilogram of body weight per day (or about 20 percent of total calories) helps preserve lean body mass and maintain metabolic rate. This amount of protein may help minimize loss of muscle mass but likely would not support the addition of lean body mass. Table 7.2 provides the amount of protein needed at each of the restricted calorie levels from table 7.1.

TABLE 7.2

Protein, Fat, and Carbohydrate Recommendations for Minimum Caloric Intake

	1,500 kcal	1,800 kcal	2,000 kcal	2,200 kcal	2,600 kcal
Protein (g)	75	90	100	110	130
Fat (g)	42	48	52	56	63
Carbohydrate (g)	206	252	283	314	378

Note: These minimum calorie levels restrict the amount of carbohydrate and should be used only during those training periods when rapid weight and fat loss will not interfere with training or performance. These diets contain 20% protein, 22 to 25% fat, and 55 to 58% carbohydrate.

Carbohydrate and Fat Balance

After you have determined your protein needs, the remaining calories should come from carbohydrate and fat (table 7.2). But one of the problems with calorie restriction at the minimum recommended level is that the athlete must make sacrifices. The choices are to restrict carbohydrate intake to prevent fat intake from being extremely low or to restrict fat intake in an effort to consume as much carbohydrate as possible. Neither situation is ideal, but the dilemma presents itself because your protein consumption must be sufficient even when you restrict calorie intake.

To keep fat intake from being extremely low, a weight-loss diet, especially one based on the minimum amount of calories recommended, should contain at least 20 to 25 percent of total calories as fat. The downside to a calorie-restricted diet containing a moderate percentage of fat is that it sacrifices carbohydrate intake to some degree. If you follow the recommendations in table 7.2, your carbohydrate intake will be a little more than 4 grams per kilogram. Normally, athletes should consume at least 5 grams of carbohydrate per kilogram of body weight so that they can fully restore muscle glycogen stores on a daily basis, but during a weight-loss diet sacrificing some carbohydrate intake may be the best option.

Why sacrifice carbohydrate more than fat? One reason is that diets containing small amounts of fat fail to satisfy hunger, which makes the diet plan difficult to follow. If a very low-fat diet is consumed over a long period, the diet may inadequately replenish intramuscular triglycerides, which are important for endurance and ultraendurance athletes. A low-fat diet may also affect the manufacture of sex-related hormones in both males and females. Wrestlers who consumed a low-fat, low-calorie diet were found to have lower testosterone levels (Strauss, Lanese, Malarkey 1985). Very low-fat diets can alter the ratio of high-density lipoproteins (good cholesterol) to low-density lipoproteins (bad cholesterol) and result in inadequate intake of fat-soluble vitamins. Some athletes may become fearful of eating fat even when they are not restricting calories. For all these reasons many nutrition professionals caution against a very low-fat weight-loss diet.

Although it may be obvious, we want to note that athletes should eliminate alcohol during periods of calorie restriction. Alcohol provides calories but not nutrients, so eliminating alcohol from the diet is an effective way to reduce calories without reducing nutrient intake.

Resistance Training

Studies of overweight adults have shown that when 10 kilograms (22 pounds) of weight is lost only through calorie restriction, approximately 2.9 kilograms (6.4 pounds) in men and 2.2 kilograms (4.8 pounds) in women is lost as fat-free mass (FFM), including some muscle mass (Garrow and Summerbell, 1995). When exercise accompanies the calorie restriction, the reduction in FFM was about 1.9 kilograms (4.2 pounds) in both genders. The conclusion that can be drawn from these studies is that the addition of exercise to a restricted calorie diet is beneficial for preserving some fat-free mass. Although these studies were not conducted in athletes, athletes should continue to exercise while they restrict caloric intake.

Those who are trying to lose weight should add or continue to perform some high-intensity, high-volume resistance exercise to preserve muscle mass and maintain metabolic rate. (See appendix A for more information on resistance training.)

Maintaining Training During Weight Loss

When athletes restrict food intake they will find it more difficult to get the nutrients that they need. A lack of calories, especially those from carbohydrate, can make maintaining a training schedule difficult. One strategy to keep your training on track is to eat small meals or snacks six times a day, with some complex carbohydrate in each. This method helps stabilize your blood sugar level and helps you feel more energetic. Another strategy is to take a rest day to replenish muscle glycogen stores a bit more.

Ultimately, low carbohydrate intake over days and weeks can reduce the ability to train. If you use the aforementioned strategies and still have trouble keeping up with your training, the best approach is to increase your calorie intake slightly by eating a greater amount of complex carbohydrate. The fiber content of complex carbohydrate helps to satisfy you, lessens your hunger, and results in a slower rise in blood glucose. Of course, a caloric increase will slow the rate of the weight loss. For that reason, substantial weight changes are best made in the off-season or early preseason, if possible, because maintaining training and performance when you are in a semistarvation state is difficult.

Personalized Caloric Restriction

So far this chapter has focused on restricting caloric intake to minimum levels that are likely to be safe and effective. Many athletes want to lose weight as rapidly as they can without losing significant lean body mass or undermining training or performance—a tall order. Athletes in sports that have weight classes (for example, wrestling, boxing), emphasize appearance (for example, bodybuilding, figure skating, ballet), or have a need for low body weight (for example, jockeying, ski jumping) are most likely to use the minimum calorie recommendations. Athletes who are expected to appear at training camp at a certain scale weight and do not have enough time to lose the weight slowly may also use the minimum calorie recommendations.

The minimum calorie recommendations are hard to follow and are too low in carbohydrate to be optimal. For those reasons, losing weight more slowly over a longer period is generally better. Slower weight loss means that the magnitude of the calorie restriction each day can be less and the amount of carbohydrate consumed can be greater. To determine how much you should restrict caloric intake daily, you need to know how many calories you normally take in and expend daily when training. This information is obtained by analyzing dietary intake and physical activity as described in chapter 3.

Athletes often apply the 500-calorie formula—reducing current food intake and increasing current physical activity to produce a 500-kilocalorie deficit each day. The 500-calorie formula can be a good starting point, but it should be modified on a case-by-case basis. Some people, especially small female athletes, find that they cannot reduce their caloric intake by even 300 kilocalories daily. Some people may be unable to increase their exercise output by 200 kilocalories over their current exercise level because they are already doing a high volume of exercise, have low fitness, or simply do not have time to exercise enough to burn that many calories. On the other hand, some athletes, particularly large-bodied males, may be consuming a large amount of calories daily just to stay in energy balance. They could safely reduce their food intake by more than 500 kilocalories and increase their energy expenditure from exercise. As always, the recommendations must be tailored to the individual.

To illustrate, we will use an example of a female collegiate tennis player who wants to lose 10 pounds (4.5 kilograms) of body fat (see table 7.3). She should do this either during the off-season or early in the preseason. Using her dietary intake and energy expenditure assessment information, she can formulate a plan that results in a calorie deficit. For example, in the off-season she could reduce her caloric intake by 150 kilocalories and increase her exercise by 150 kilocalories each day. Doing this would require only simple changes such as not having chips at lunch and walking at a moderate pace for about 30 minutes each day. With a daily caloric deficit of 300 kilocalories, she would lose 10 pounds (4.5 kilograms) in about 17 weeks.

TABLE 7.3

Daily Food Intake and Activity Adjustments for a Female Collegiate Tennis Player to Lose 10 Pounds (4.5 Kilograms)

	Off-season (17 weeks)	Early preseason (13 weeks)	Late preseason (10 weeks)*	Competitive season (12 weeks)*
Weight-loss plan to reduce 10 lb (4.5 kg) body fat	Decrease daily food intake by 150 kcal and increase daily physical activity by 150 kcal	Increase exercise by 500 kcal daily** but increase food intake by only 100 kcal daily	None	None
Total calorie deficit	300 kcal daily	400 kcal daily	None	None
Time to achieve 10 lb weight loss	17 weeks	12 1/2 weeks		

This example assumes that metabolic rate does not change.
*To maintain performance, weight loss is typically not recommended during this time.
**Assumes that the athlete has the fitness to increase exercise to this extent.

If she chooses not to lose body fat during the off-season, another option is to lose 10 pounds (4.5 kilograms) early in the preseason. When preseason training starts, energy expenditure through physical activity goes up considerably when compared with the off-season. In this example, when the athlete returns to rigorous training she increases her energy expenditure by 500 kilocalories per day. Usually, when she returns to training she increases her food intake by 500 kilocalories daily and maintains her weight. If she wants to lose 10 pounds (4.5 kilograms), she can create a daily calorie deficit of 400 kilocalories by increasing her food intake by 100 kilocalories daily. Because her early preseason training period is 13 weeks long, she should be able to reach her goal of losing 10 pounds (4.5 kilograms) within this period. By including resistance exercise as part of her training and conditioning, she should be able to protect against the loss of muscle mass while losing body fat. Timing of meals and snacks is critical in this preseason example because she needs to support her training with sufficient energy and nutrients.

Either plan will help her meet her goal. In the off-season she has more time and can slightly decrease food intake and slightly increase activity each day to achieve a slow, sustained loss of body fat. If she waits until preseason training begins, she has less time so the daily changes have to be more substantial. A return to rigorous training means that the intensity and duration of exercise accounts for most of the caloric deficit. This example assumes that her fitness and conditioning is sufficient to tolerate the rigorous training.

The off-season and the early preseason are usually the best times to attempt weight loss. Losing weight later in the preseason may put the athlete at a competitive disadvantage to athletes who are not restricting their caloric intake. As the competitive season nears, the focus should be on maintaining body composition and peak performance. As you can see, planning is essential to losing weight without undermining training, performance, or health.

Supplemental Exercise

Supplemental exercise plays an important role in helping athletes lose weight as body fat. If you increase your exercise and do not increase your food intake, you will create a calorie deficit. The frequency, intensity, and duration of exercise, especially prolonged aerobic exercise, can create a substantial caloric deficit. Resistance training typically creates only a mild calorie deficit, but as noted previously resistance training is essential to minimizing the loss of lean body mass and lessening the reduction in metabolic rate.

You must be careful about adding too much supplemental exercise because you do not want to overtrain. You should also add the right kinds of supplemental exercise (aerobic or resistance) so that you do not undermine the training and conditioning plan that you already have in place. You may be already training vigorously and be unable to realistically increase your daily volume of high-intensity exercise. Instead, the supplemental exercise that you add to help burn body fat stores will likely be moderate in intensity. In many cases the best approach is to increase daily physical activity by walking instead of driving a car, by climbing stairs, and by participating in active leisure pastimes, all of which contribute to a daily energy deficit.

Psychological Strategies for Losing Fat

There is more to losing weight than just adjusting your dietary intake and exercise output. Psychological factors should not be overlooked. Fat loss usually involves restriction, and restricting something as essential as food is a powerful psychological challenge. Restrained eating sometimes leads to binge eating because the restriction of food involves intense emotions. One strategy to help you overcome this barrier is to restrict food intake only moderately. When deprivation is considerable, the temptation to splurge may become irresistible.

Another powerful issue is emotional eating. Food intake can be temporarily comforting when you are sad, anxious, or stressed. If a person uses food as an emotional comfort, food restriction can be psychologically uncomfortable because a weight-loss diet is a form of physical and emotional stress. If you struggle with emotional eating, stop before you engage in any unplanned eating and ask yourself what is motivating your actions. If stress is the underlying motive, identify ways other than eating to address the stress.

Certain foods that you find enjoyable can trigger eating. For example, many people enjoy chocolate and eliminating it would cause them psychological stress. The key is to identify trigger foods and determine an acceptable way to handle them. No two people are alike. Some people do best by eliminating the trigger food altogether when they are trying to restrict calories. That way they are not tempted. Others do best when their plan allows for limited portions of the trigger food so that they can consume it on a near daily basis and do not have to fight their craving.

Evaluation and Reassessment

Any plan will likely need adjustments. Because the goal is to drop weight but not strength, power, or endurance, objective measurements must be made to evaluate the effectiveness of the diet plan. Losing body fat takes time, so evaluating the results may not be realistic until four weeks after beginning the plan. At that time reassessment of scale weight, body composition, metabolic rate, and measures of strength, power, speed, or endurance provide objective measurements for determining whether the diet plan should remain unchanged or be adjusted in some way. But if it is clear at any time that training cannot be maintained or that performance is declining, changes need to be made immediately.

For example, a male boxer creates a plan to lose 15 pounds (6.8 kilograms) to achieve a weight that he feels is competitive with other boxers in his weight class. His weight-loss plan includes increased energy expenditure through training and restricted food intake. After four weeks, a reassessment shows that he is reducing scale weight and body fat, and maintaining his strength and endurance. His plan is working. Over the next month, however, he finds it difficult to maintain his training and performance. His second reassessment (eight weeks after the original assessment) shows that he is not losing weight and body fat as he expected and that his strength and endurance is declining. The plan that was working four weeks earlier is no longer working. He needs to make adjustments.

He may be able to detect some of the problems by examining the reassessment information. For example, if his resting metabolic rate is lower, his caloric restriction may be too severe. A dietary assessment may show that his nutrient intake is consistently low. Thus, the effects of taking in too little carbohydrate and insufficient vitamins and minerals over time may have caught up with him. These problems are not always evident immediately, so a plan that appeared to be working at four weeks may need to be revised later on.

In this case, the athlete may need to increase caloric intake by a small amount to make sure that the food restriction is not causing a decrease in metabolic rate. The foods consumed could also be altered so that they are nutrient dense and provide a large amount of nutrients in proportion to their caloric content. Carbohydrate intake could be increased to provide the fuel needed to train and maintain strength, power, and endurance. By completing step 4 of the four steps to achieving optimal performance weight, the athlete can get back on track.

Weighing In on Water Weight

It is no secret that athletes can lower their body weight by shedding body water. Likewise, it is no secret that some athletes have died doing so. The issue then is not whether you can do it but whether you should do it. And if you choose to do it, what methods are safe? Knowing the benefits of proper hydration and the risks of dehydration on performance and health are important as you make decisions about controlling water weight, particularly before weigh-ins.

Although avoiding dehydration is a challenge for most athletes, a handful must also be concerned about hyperhydration—excessive body water. Hyperhydration can lead to low blood sodium, known as hyponatremia, which can be fatal. Humans are essentially water organisms, so missteps in the management of body water are not limited to negative effects on performance. Water-related mishaps affect health along a continuum that ranges from mild to severe to fatal.

Between 40 and 70 percent of your weight is water. No matter what the exact percentage is for you, the point is that water is a substantial component of the body's scale weight. Clearly then, water plays a critical role in the functioning of the body and offers an obvious target for manipulation by athletes who need to make weight.

Dehydration and Water Balance

Dehydration is an excess loss of body water, often defined as a loss of 2 percent or more of body weight as water. Percent water lost is estimated by comparing scale weight before and after exercise and converting that difference into a percentage. For example, if an athlete begins exercise weighing 167 pounds (76 kilograms) and his postexercise weight is 162 pounds (73.6 kilograms), then he has lost 3 percent (5 lb ÷ 167 or 2.4 kg ÷ 76) of body weight as water.

Water is lost from the body in four ways: (1) ventilation (breathing), (2) nonsweat skin losses (such as water emanating from pores to keep the skin from drying and cracking), (3) sweating, and (4) excretion, primarily through urine but also in feces. Water is provided to the body in three ways: (1) beverages, (2) food, and (3) as a byproduct of (H_2O) chemical reactions. Under normal circumstances the body can easily maintain fluid balance because it can counterbalance water loss with water intake.

Water balance is not difficult to achieve under nonstressful conditions. For example, a person who is sitting in a 70 degrees Fahrenheit (21 degrees Celsius) room loses only a small amount of water, which eating and drinking can easily restore. Should the person consume more water than was lost, the body would become slightly overhydrated and temporarily out of equilibrium. In response, the body would increase the amount of water excreted as urine to bring body water back into balance. Should the body become slightly dehydrated, then the sensation of thirst would signal to the person to drink some fluid. In these ways, the body can easily maintain fluid balance in nonstressful conditions.

Exercise generates heat, causing stress and presenting a challenge to maintaining fluid equilibrium. For example, large amounts of water can be lost in sweat, especially when exercise is performed in the heat. At the same time that water is being lost through sweat, water intake may be limited because high-intensity exercise slows water absorption from the intestines. Simply stated, when sweat losses are substantial during exercise, water intake cannot keep up with water loss and the body becomes dehydrated. Note that athletes who train and perform in the water, such as swimmers and water polo players, also sweat to dissipate body heat; therefore, dehydration in these athletes should not be overlooked.

Stressful conditions created by exercise, particularly in the heat, simply overwhelm the body's usual regulatory mechanisms—urine volume and thirst. At first, the degree of dehydration is minor, but it becomes more pronounced as the body continues to lose water through sweat and as water intake fails to keep pace.

Effects of Dehydration on Performance

Environmental heat reduces work or exercise output even when a person is well hydrated. In other words, you cannot work or exercise as hard in the heat as you can in temperate conditions. Dehydration also decreases work and exercise output. In a study done in the California desert, an environmental temperature of 43 degrees Celsius (109.4 degrees Fahrenheit) or a 2.5 percent decrease in body water resulted in a decline in work output of about 25 percent. When the subjects experienced both conditions, the decline in work output was 50 percent. The effect of dehydration and a hot environment is additive, meaning that each condition affects performance independent of the other.

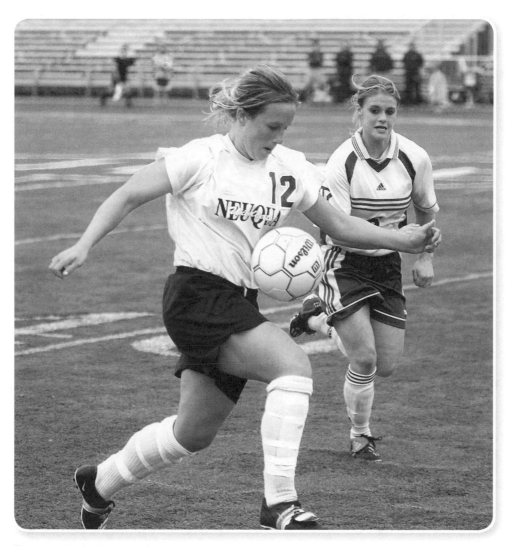

To prevent a decline in performance, soccer players and other athletes must be careful to replenish the water lost through sweat.

Most dehydration research has been conducted in aerobic athletes—such as distance runners, cyclists, and those in ball sports—in temperate to hot climates. Table 8.1 lists some of the effects of dehydration on aerobic performance. Research studies have consistently shown that a fluid loss of as little as 2 percent of body weight negatively affects aerobic performance in these conditions. Studies have also shown that the greater the degree of dehydration, the greater the degree of performance decline. A limited number of studies suggest that dehydration causes cognitive performance to decline, which could result in mental or strategic mistakes. Thus, athletes must stay well hydrated.

Far fewer studies have been conducted about the effects of dehydration on anaerobic performance, such as occurs in wrestling or weightlifting.

TABLE 8.1

Effects of Dehydration on Aerobic Performance

Sport	Degree of dehydration*	Effect on performance
Basketball	2%	Movement slows, shooting is less accurate, and attention declines. Performance continues to decline as the degree of dehydration increases.
Distance cycling	2.5%	On a two-hour ride with hills, power output for hill climbing declines.
1,500 m run	2%	Running time increases by about 3%.
5,000 or 10,000 m run	2%	Running time increases by about 5%.
Soccer	1.5–2%	Playing ability and fitness declines; perceived exertion increases.

*Percent loss of body weight as water.

Data from Armstrong, Costill, Fink, 1985; Baker, Conroy, Kenney, 2007; Baker, Dougherty, Chow, et al., 2007; Ebert, Martin, Bullock, et al., 2007; Edwards, Mann, Marfell-Jones, et al., 2007.

These studies have shown that fluid losses between 3 and 5 percent of body weight do not appear to affect either muscle strength or anaerobic performance (Maughan 2003). But dehydration may affect cognitive performance. The degree of dehydration also affects health. Wrestling governing bodies have made rule changes to prevent wrestlers from using dehydration as a weight-loss method.

Dangers of Dehydration

Many athletes make the mistake of overlooking the health risks of dehydration to focus on the weight loss that they can achieve by reducing body water. Remember, however, that wrestlers usually do not die on the mat; they die in the training room as they are trying to reduce scale weight rapidly through loss of body water, before they even have a chance to compete. Similarly, athletes collapse on the training field because of heat illnesses related to elevated body temperature, which can be caused by dehydration.

Dehydration as a Weight-Loss Method

Those who intentionally use dehydration as a weight-loss method must be aware that they are flirting with danger. Two major factors associated with a life-threatening outcome are the degree (how much) and rapidity (how fast) of dehydration. The athlete at greatest risk for potentially fatal medical problems is the one who is already dehydrated and tries to lose more body water rapidly. Using large and rapid water loss to attain a particular scale weight is known as cutting weight. Boxers, bodybuilders, jockeys, lightweight rowers, martial artists, and wrestlers are the athletes most likely to cut weight, although rule changes in wrestling have helped reduce the amount of water weight that competitors may lose.

Because the time to lose weight before weigh-in is short, these athletes reduce the component of body weight that they can affect most quickly—body water. The methods that they use to cut weight include fluid restriction, fasting, reducing sodium intake, excessive exercise in the heat or while wearing extra clothing, diuretics, laxatives, vomiting, and sitting in a sauna. Athletes commonly employ more than one of these methods and, if they are desperate, all of them.

For many years losing large amounts of weight before weigh-in was a badge of honor for wrestlers. Until the late 1990s, 40 percent of collegiate wrestlers routinely lost 10 to 20 pounds (4.5 to 9 kilograms) each week throughout the season. In 1997 three collegiate wrestlers died because of large, rapid reductions in weight, primarily as water. These deaths prompted rule changes such as a shorter time between weigh-in and competition and measurement of the specific gravity of urine (a measure of dehydration). Such changes have reduced the amount and severity of weight loss by wrestlers. But other sports, such as the martial arts, certify weight 20 to 30 hours before competition, a practice that allows athletes to lose larger amounts of water weight because they have more time to replenish with food and fluid before the match.

Dehydration and Diuretics

One method for inducing water loss is the use of a diuretic, which increases urine output. Powerful diuretics are commonly prescribed to those with high blood pressure, edema (swelling because of water retention), and congestive heart failure, to rid the body of excess water. Some athletes use diuretics as an ill-conceived technique to reduce scale weight, and some bodybuilders use them to remove body water so that muscles are more clearly defined. Because these are inappropriate uses of the medications, these athletes may obtain prescription diuretics illegally or use over-the-counter supplements that contain compounds with diuretic properties.

The Water Weight-Loss Myth

Many athletes may have been told that loss of water weight is not a problem until it exceeds 10 pounds (4.5 kilograms) or 5 percent of body weight. Although more medical problems occur as dehydration becomes more severe, it is a myth that a threshold marks the border between safe and unsafe water weight loss. No one can identify with certainty the point at which an athlete is entering the danger zone. Water and electrolyte (such as sodium or potassium) balance can shift quickly, and an athlete who loses water weight rapidly can go from normal body function to a life-threatening condition within hours.

The usual mechanism for most diuretics is to inhibit the reabsorption of sodium in the kidney, which keeps water from being reabsorbed. Some diuretics also deplete potassium, magnesium, and calcium along with the sodium and water. Use of powerful diuretics increases the risk for dehydration and electrolyte imbalance, which can lead to medical problems such as cardiac arrest. The manufacturers of prescription diuretics warn physicians to regulate the dosage carefully to avoid rapid or substantial loss of fluid and electrolytes and to discontinue use if excessive water loss occurs. Thus, an athlete who uses a prescription diuretic for weight loss is attempting to do what the manufacturer has warned against.

Taking a fast-acting diuretic or a higher dose of a diuretic than would normally be prescribed for a person's body weight are particularly dangerous practices. Some of the deaths associated with prescription diuretic use have been in bodybuilders who have taken furosemide (originally Lasix but now available as a generic), a powerful and fast-acting diuretic. On the day of a competition, some bodybuilders feel that they are holding water, a level of extracellular water that may obscure muscle definition (a criterion used to judge contestants).

Furosemide results in a decrease in extracellular water, but it causes excess loss of potassium, magnesium, and calcium in the urine. In a matter of hours, blood levels of these electrolytes can become too low, and bodybuilders may faint, cramp up while posing, develop an irregular heartbeat, or die of cardiac arrest. In many cases the symptoms come on quickly and without warning.

Some athletes use natural diuretics, which are herbals that increase urine output. These are sold as dietary supplements. More than 200 herbs are known to have a diuretic effect. Supplements and "diet teas" contain various combinations of substances including birch leaf, goldenrod, juniper berry, and licorice root. Combining several herbals with diuretic properties can produce the same effect as a prescription diuretic.

Athletes may believe that herbal diuretics are safer than prescription ones. Safety depends to a large degree on the dose of the active ingredient, but knowing the dose of an herbal supplement is often difficult. The dose may not be listed on the label, the product may contain more or less of the diuretic than is stated, or the product may be contaminated with other compounds. Herbal supplements are not well regulated by the Food and Drug Administration and should be used with caution.

Influence of Dehydration on Body Temperature

A critical problem when exercising or competing in the heat is hyperthermia, which is an abnormally elevated body temperature. Normal body temperature is 98.6 degrees Fahrenheit (37 degrees Celsius), although minor variations occur among individuals and in any given individual based on time of day. Studies have shown that dehydration in athletes who perform aerobic exercise in temperate, warm, or hot climates increases the risk for hyperthermia. This increased risk is associated with the degree of dehydration. In other words, a 2 percent loss of body weight from fluid loss is a risk for elevated body temperature, but a 3 percent loss is a greater risk.

Exercise results in the internal production of heat and raises body temperature. The body responds to an increase in internal temperature by sweating to dissipate heat from the body. When sweat evaporates from the surface of the skin, heat is transported away from the body. The benefit of sweating is that it cools the temperature of the body, but a disadvantage is that the body loses water in the process.

Athletes may face additional conditions that decrease the ability of the body to cool itself. When humidity is high the air is more saturated with water, so the sweat on the surface of the skin does not evaporate. Uniforms and sauna suits also obstruct the evaporation of sweat. In such cases, body water is lost, but the usual benefit of sweating—cooling—does not occur.

The loss of large amounts of water as sweat also reduces blood volume, which negatively affects body temperature. Sweating is not the only way that skin is involved in dissipating heat. Heat is also transported by the blood to the surface of the skin where the heat can be transferred to the air. When blood volume is low, blood flow to the skin is in competition with blood flow to exercising muscle so heat dissipation though the skin decreases. Extra clothing or sauna suits further prevent the dissipation of heat.

Physiological responses to exercise in the heat vary widely among athletes. Some are far more heat tolerant than others. Dehydration and rising body temperature can lead to varying forms of heat illness, including heat cramps, heat exhaustion, and heat stroke. Heat illness results in declines in performance, but the critical and more immediate issue is the effect on health.

Heat cramps in muscles that are being exercised to the point of fatigue are likely the result of rapid and excessive loss of fluid and sodium in sweat. Well-documented case studies of both football and tennis players have shown that those who are "heavy, salty sweaters" experience debilitating heat cramps. Such athletes must use a highly individualized hydration strategy to minimize excessive losses of body water and sodium and to reduce the risks to health and performance.

Heat exhaustion is related to low blood volume resulting from a significant loss of body water. It may also involve excessive loss of electrolytes (for example, sodium and potassium). An athlete who experiences heat exhaustion becomes fatigued, sweats profusely, and feels thirsty. If the athlete does not stop exercising and seek medical attention (typically ingesting salty water or carbohydrate-electrolyte sports drink by mouth or a saline solution by IV), his or her medical condition will continue to decline. Athletes can decrease their risk for heat exhaustion by avoiding dehydration as much as possible (by consuming fluids during exercise) and by training in the heat 10 to 14 days before training camp or competition to help acclimatize the body.

Heat stroke is a medical emergency because it is life threatening. Heat stroke occurs when a person's internal temperature exceeds 104 degrees

Fahrenheit (40 degrees Celsius). This condition affects the central nervous system and threatens the functioning of major organs such as the brain, heart, and kidneys. Primary factors in heat stroke are strenuous exercise in hot and humid conditions, poor physical fitness, and lack of acclimatization to heat. Large-bodied football players who show up in poor physical condition at preseason training camps held in hot and humid conditions or recreational athletes who have not trained in the heat for a long event such as a marathon are two examples of athletes who are at high risk. In 1997 three collegiate wrestlers died from heat stroke. They used a combination of extreme methods, including severe dehydration, to lose body weight.

However, well-trained, well-acclimatized, lean athletes can also experience heat stroke even when they are properly hydrated, so do not assume that heat stroke cannot happen to you. Athletes should try to avoid or minimize dehydration as much as possible during exercise in the heat, not only as a way to decrease the risk for heat stroke and other heat-related illnesses but also because being well hydrated offers performance and health benefits.

Food and Water Manipulation for Rapid Weight Loss

Athletes who need to have their weight certified often ask whether they can safely manipulate food and water intake in the 24 hours before weigh-in. The diet-related strategies commonly used are restricting sodium, food, or fluid intake one or two days before weigh-in or a bodybuilding contest.

Any practice employed to cut weight may be unsafe, but temporarily restricting sodium intake is the least likely of the three to cause serious harm to performance and health. Sodium is associated with water retention. When sodium is consumed in food nearly 100 percent of the sodium is absorbed. Water will also be temporarily retained until the body can reestablish sodium and water balance by excreting excess sodium and water in the urine.

When sodium is temporarily increased in the blood, which may occur after consumption of a salty food or meal, water is pulled into the blood from the cells. Blood volume temporarily increases, the cells become slightly dehydrated, and a complex hormonal response eventually drives the person to drink more fluid. Fluid intake offsets the temporary increase in blood sodium and restores water balance. Similarly, a decrease in blood sodium decreases the amount of water in the blood, but blood sodium can decrease only slightly before the risk of heat illness increases.

Restricting dietary sodium can result in loss of body water through urine as the body tries to reestablish sodium and water balance. Reducing sodium intake to very low amounts (for example, 1,000 to 1,500 milligrams daily) would likely result in a loss of about 600 milliliters (2.5 cups) of water on the first day or about 1.25 pounds (.57 kilogram) of scale weight. Over a seven-day period the total loss of water weight from substantial sodium reduction is likely to be about 3 pounds (1.4 kilograms).

Note that a 1,000 to 1,500 milligram sodium diet is extremely low in sodium. Thus, many familiar and convenient foods usually consumed would have to be temporarily excluded. Eating in fast-food outlets or other restaurants would be difficult. As a short-term strategy, reducing sodium intake to very low amounts can result in a temporary loss of fluid and a loss of 1 to 3 pounds (.45 to 1.4 kilograms) of water weight. The short-term restriction of sodium is not likely to affect health negatively because the body has a large reserve of sodium in bones. But sodium restriction is not useful as a long-term strategy to lose body fat.

Restricting food intake one to two days before weigh-in is a short-term starvation state to which the body can adapt. A few immediate health problems are likely to occur, such as headaches, irritability, light-headedness, and a reduced ability to concentrate. Substantial performance-related problems can develop, including the depletion of liver and muscle glycogen and the breakdown of muscle protein. A 24- or 48-hour fast might result in a loss of 1 to 3 pounds (0.45 to 1.4 kilograms) of weight (depending on body size), but about two-thirds of the weight lost will be water, glycogen, and protein.

Restricting water intake, even for a day or two, is a dangerous practice and is not recommended. Water restriction is particularly harmful to the tissues that contain a large proportion of water. Blood is about 90 percent water, and muscle and organs typically contain 70 to 80 percent water. One cup of water weighs about 240 grams, or 0.5 pound. When water is restricted the body compensates by reducing the amount of urine excreted, so water restriction is not likely to produce a large loss of scale weight. But it immediately affects blood, muscle, and organ function and has the potential to damage the kidneys.

Athletes who choose to reduce water weight before weigh-in should begin fluid consumption immediately after weight is certified. The amount of fluid that a person can tolerate will vary, but the goal is to get as close as possible to 100 percent restoration of hydration. The degree to which dehydration can be reversed depends on the length of time until competition, which may be as short as one to two hours. Some ways to tell whether hydration status is improving include greater urine volume, lighter urine color, and less thirst.

If you have restricted intake of food and water before weigh-in, consume a carbohydrate-containing beverage as soon as your weight is certified. Such a beverage helps restore fluid balance, replenish muscle and liver glycogen, and increase blood sugar level, which will help you feel more energetic.

Overhydration and Hyponatremia

Most of this chapter has focused on fluid imbalance because of dehydration, but fluid imbalance can also result from overhydration. In the past, athletes were encouraged to drink as much as possible. Although this advice was intended to help athletes prevent dehydration, it had unintended consequences. Some distance athletes, such as slow marathon runners and Ironman competitors, drank so much water that the amount of sodium in their blood became diluted. Hyponatremia, the medical term for low blood sodium, is a potentially fatal condition, especially when sodium drops rapidly and stays low.

The prevailing advice today is to match fluid intake with fluid loss. During prolonged endurance exercise, athletes should consume some salty foods or beverages to make sure that their blood sodium does not drop too low. Those who sweat heavily or sweat a lot of salt may need to drink a specially formulated electrolyte beverage to help replace significant electrolyte losses. To prevent both hyponatremia and dehydration, the athlete must develop an individualized plan for proper fluid and sodium intake during exercise.

Preventing Dehydration

Athletes who train or compete in hot or humid conditions will have difficulty preventing dehydration because they will be losing body water faster than they can replace it. Part of the reason is that a time lag occurs between the loss of body water, the changing concentration of sodium in the blood, and the hormonal and central nervous system stimuli that create the sensation of thirst.

Another reason is that the amount of fluid that can be absorbed from the intestinal tract may be less than the amount of water that is being lost.

Hydration Assessment

Many athletes are not adequately hydrated when they begin a training session or competition, in part because they do not rehydrate adequately after exercising. A quick way to evaluate your daily hydration status is to determine your thirst, weight, and urine color first thing every morning. Although these assessments are remarkably simple, they are good indicators of hydration status.

If you are thirsty when you wake up, then your body is telling you that it needs more fluid. Thirst, one of the ways that your body drives you to drink, is a message that you are not properly hydrated. Another way to tell whether you drank enough fluid over the previous 24 hours is to look at the color of your urine. If you are adequately hydrated your urine will be a very light yellow color. If you are dehydrated your urine will be a darker yellow. Finally, after you have urinated take a scale weight and compare it to your weight from the previous morning. If your weight is more than 0.5 percent less, you have probably not rehydrated adequately. For example, if your weight yesterday morning was 154 pounds (70 kilograms) but your weight this morning is 153 pounds (69.5 kilograms), then you are probably dehydrated.

Although you may drink a certain amount of fluid, not all of that fluid will be absorbed or absorbed rapidly. Keep in mind that fluid can be absorbed at a rate of about 4 to 6 ounces (120 to 180 milliliters) every 15 minutes. If you have ever drank too much too fast and then felt the fluid sloshing around your stomach, you have experienced some of the effects of slow absorption.

High-intensity exercise, especially in the heat, may slow fluid absorption from both the stomach and the intestine. Depending on the sport, drinking large amounts of fluid during competition may be difficult. For example, time-outs and substitutions may give basketball or soccer players a chance to consume water or other beverages, but the amount of fluid that they can consume will not likely match the amount that they lose during play.

Most athletes cannot prevent dehydration during exercise, but they can reduce its severity. Remember that hydration is on a continuum. Problems can become more severe as you become more dehydrated. Each athlete needs to develop a short-term plan for fluid intake, and possibly sodium intake, during exercise and a long-term plan for overall water and electrolyte balance.

To create a personalized hydration plan, you should estimate how much you sweat. To determine your sweat rate, complete the following steps:

1. Take your body weight nude or in minimal clothing before and after you exercise (Note: do not urinate before taking your postexercise weight).
2. Measure how much fluid you consumed during the exercise.
3. Measure how many minutes you exercised.
4. Calculate your sweat rate using table 8.2.
5. Repeat under various environmental conditions (for example, heat, humidity).

Table 8.2 outlines how to calculate sweat rate. Record pre- and postexercise weights so that you can calculate change in body weight. You must account for any fluid that you consumed during exercise for the calculations to be correct. Column E is the total amount of sweat lost in milliliters. By dividing sweat loss by the number of minutes that you exercised, you can calculate your sweat rate, which is given in milliliters of sweat lost per minute.

In table 8.2, two examples illustrate how to calculate sweat rate. Both athletes lost more than 30 milliliters (1 ounce) of fluid per minute. In one hour of exercising in the heat, each would lose more than 1,800 milliliters, which is equivalent to 60 ounces, or about 7 1/2 cups. The challenge for these athletes is to consume during exercise as close to the amount lost as possible, keeping in mind that fluid can be absorbed at about 4 to 6 ounces (120 to 180 milliliters) every 15 minutes.

Precisely measuring the amount of sodium being lost during exercise is difficult, but there are two general ways to tell whether sodium losses are large.

TABLE 8.2

Calculating Sweat Rate

A	B	C	D	E	F	G
Preexercise body weight	Immediate[a] postexercise body weight	Change in body weight (A – B)	Fluid consumed during exercise	Sweat loss (C + D)[b]	Exercise time	Sweat rate (E / F)
70 kg	68.5 kg	1.5 kg (1,500 g) [b]	480 ml	1,980 ml	60 min	33 ml/min
157 lb	154 lb	3 lb (1,364 g)[c]	2 cups (480 ml)[d]	1,844 ml	60 min	31 ml/min

[a]Do not urinate before taking a scale weight.
[b]1 g change in weight = 1 ml of fluid.
[c]To convert lb to g, divide weight in lb by 2.2 and multiply by 1,000.
[d]1 cup = 8 oz or 240 ml; 1 oz = 30 ml.
Adapted, by permission, from B. Murray, 1996, "Determining sweat rate," *Sports Science Exchange*, 9(63 Supplement):4.

Check for evidence of salt accumulation on your skin or clothing (on hatband, bandana, shirt, or socks). If salt crystals or a gritty white film is present, you are considered a salty sweater. You should also measure the amount of sweat that you lose. A loss of more than 4 liters of sweat (approximately 8.5 lb or 3.8 kg body weight) in a day typically results in substantial loss of sodium. If either of these conditions is present, then sodium replacement during exercise is usually recommended.

Sodium replenishment during exercise is usually accomplished by consuming a sports beverage that has more sodium than usual or by taking sodium supplements. Because excessive sodium intake can have negative medical effects, you may want to work with a physician or sports dietitian to determine the amount of sodium that would be best for you if you are a salty sweater. Many athletes also lightly salt their food or consume a salty snack such as pretzels after exercise to make sure that they replace some of the sodium lost during exercise. The goal is to match sodium intake with sodium loss.

To assess whether your plan is working, you should monitor the color of your urine, take morning pre- and postexercise weights on the scale while wearing little or no clothing, and be aware of thirst. You should adjust your plan based on environmental conditions.

Sizing Up Supplement Use

In times past, foods were easily distinguished from supplements, just as foods were easily distinguished from drugs. Not so today. Besides choosing foods to eat, you must make decisions about supplements, some of which have druglike effects. Changing weight and body composition by adjusting food intake takes time and effort every day. Muscle-building and fat-loss supplements are appealing because most are touted to help you achieve your goals more quickly, with less effort, and independent of your diet. Some athletes are not attentive to their diets and hope to make up for dietary shortcomings with supplements. Even athletes who are diligent about their food intake may look to supplements to help them find a competitive edge. Most athletes have questions or concerns about dietary supplements.

Surveys report that athletes in many sports engage in substantial use of dietary supplements. Estimates are that 75 percent of elite athletes take at least one dietary supplement routinely and that many take several daily. Although use of supplements by collegiate athletes is less extensive than use by professional athletes, most collegians try at least one supplement over the course of their college athletic careers. As many as one-third of all high school athletes consume a dietary supplement, although the prevalence is highest in football players and wrestlers. Frequent dietary supplement use by athletes in general, and elite athletes in particular, may result in social pressure on athletes to consume dietary supplements.

But there is no substitute for a proper diet. You should have an optimal training and performance diet in place before you consider dietary supplements. Then you will need to decide whether, and how, you want to take dietary supplements. The intention of this chapter is to provide unbiased information about supplements that will help you make an informed decision.

Rather than succumb to social pressure or sales-pitch pressure from those who sell supplements, you need to determine for yourself the health and performance risks and benefits of supplement use. You also risk your money if you buy ineffective supplements. In the end, you must decide whether the risks are worth the benefits. After all, the supplements will be going into your body.

Note that studies of dietary supplements are usually conducted in adults; therefore, most health professionals do not recommend dietary supplement use by children and adolescents. In addition, some supplement products contain compounds that are banned substances, and their use will cause athletes to test positive and be subject to penalties. Be aware of the regulations issued by the governing body of your sport. And always check with your physician before taking any dietary supplement.

Defining Supplements

In the United States, the legal definition for a dietary supplement is a vitamin, mineral, herb, botanical, amino acid, metabolite, constituent, extract, or a combination of any of these ingredients. Many products on the market may be thought of as supplements because the word *supplement* means "to add to." But some products, such as carbohydrate powders and gels and meal replacement beverages, are better described as substitutes rather than supplements because they are convenient alternatives to foods or meals.

Viewpoints on Supplementation

Professionals in sport-related fields and athletes embrace various philosophies about supplement use. Discrete categorizations of the opinions of professionals and athletes in certain sports are the result. For example, health professionals are often described as being antisupplement. Bodybuilders are typically thought of as being prosupplement. In reality, most people involved in athletics hold the same general philosophy—food first. After a proper diet is in place, they look at the need for supplementation. This is the point where philosophies begin to differ.

Health-related professionals, such as physicians and sports dietitians, tend to emphasize safety and effectiveness because they honor a basic medical principle—first, do no harm. This issue includes a critical ethical component because a harmful supplement harms the health of the athlete, not the person recommending it. Health professionals therefore recommend only those supplements scientifically shown to be safe and effective.

Most athletes are also concerned about supplement safety, but they have a different ethical issue because the risk and the benefit accrue to the same person. In other words, the person who makes the decision to take a supplement is the same person who reaps the benefits or suffers the consequences. Some athletes are risk takers. They may adopt the approach that supplements probably will not hurt and might help. Such a philosophy does not pose an ethical issue for the individual, but the idea that a substance "probably will not hurt" is beyond the ethical limits of many health professionals.

What about the people who sell supplements? Most people assume that the first priority for those who sell supplement is sales, which translates to profits. Those who sell supplements may fall anywhere on the ethical continuum. They range from those who refuse to sell products that they consider unsafe to people like the head of a now-defunct supplement company who, fellow employees said, wadded up and threw away customer complaints of supplements that had caused heart attacks, strokes, and seizures (Blumberg, 2005).

Athletes in some sports are more likely than others to focus on dietary supplements that may change body composition. For example, bodybuilders tend to look closely at supplements because the body is essentially the sport. The body is judged individually and compared with others, so besides following a well-planned training and diet program, bodybuilders often consider dietary supplements to provide a competitive edge. Similarly, dietary supplements that promote fat or water weight loss may be appealing to athletes in sports that have weight categories such as boxing and wrestling. After their weight is certified, these athletes benefit from being strong and well conditioned—performance attributes supported by months of proper training and diet. In the end nearly everyone has the same general philosophy—food first—but philosophies vary about whether, and which, supplements should be taken.

Safety and Effectiveness

Many consumers believe that if a dietary supplement is for sale, then it must be safe and effective. This belief is unfounded. The law that regulates dietary supplements does not ensure their safety or effectiveness. The consumer is responsible for determining whether a supplement is generally safe and effective. No supplement is guaranteed to be 100 percent safe, so the guiding principle is the risk-to-benefit ratio. The vast majority of supplements are unproven in their capacity to increase muscle mass or decrease body fat, so for most supplements the risk is typically greater than the benefit.

Over-the-counter medications (for example, aspirin) must meet strict quality control measures including verification that each pill contains only the ingredients and amounts stated on the label. Known as good manufacturing practice (GMP), these rules are rigorously applied to prescription and over-the-counter medications and offer the highest degree of quality control against contamination with other substances. Unfortunately, when dietary supplements became regulated in the United States in 1994, GMP was not required. This circumstance led to various degrees of quality control. Supplements were sold without a listing of ingredients or amounts on the label. Athletes thus faced a significant problem because some supplements were contaminated with banned substances. Some supplements contained higher doses than were shown on the label, a particular problem with herbal supplements. Purity was not guaranteed.

The Marketing of Supplements

The sheer number of supplements sold, especially over the Internet, makes it impossible to regulate all supplement advertising. Government resources are limited, so the focus is on a handful of supplements and manufacturers who represent the greatest risk for consumers. Most false marketing claims go unchallenged. In a study of 300 advertisements for weight-loss supplements, 40 percent of the ads included a claim that was false. Another 15 percent made claims that could not be substantiated, so the likelihood was high that they were false. Although few studies have been conducted, a reasonable assumption is that at least half of the marketing claims made for dietary supplements for the purpose of weight loss are false. Simply stated, there are no guarantees that the claims made in advertisements of any dietary supplements for athletes are factual.

Dietary supplements are frequently marketed directly to athletes. Someone closely associated with your team or sport may pressure you to buy a particular supplement. Those selling supplements do not offer unbiased information. The information may not necessarily be false, but a person who stands to benefit financially from your supplement purchase is biased. The prospect of financial gain is a powerful motivator and can cause people to put less emphasis on proved effectiveness. Before you decide to take a supplement, find unbiased sources of information about its safety and effectiveness. This book is one source. Health professionals who do not sell supplements, such as most physicians and registered dietitians and some pharmacists, are other sources of unbiased information about safety and effectiveness. Be sure to ask and answer several basic questions about every dietary supplement that you are thinking about taking: *Is it legal? Is it ethical? Is it safe? Is it effective?*

Contamination of dietary supplements was such a concern that in 2004 the National Football League (NFL) began a supplement certification program carried out by an independent testing agency so that its players could be confident that the certified supplements did not contain banned substances. When choosing supplements, one protection for athletes is to buy only those that are certified. The label will contain a certification logo indicating that the product has met GMP standards similar to those used to produce medications. Unfortunately, because of the high cost of certification, few manufacturers have had their products evaluated. Athletes should also be aware that many supplements available for purchase in the United States are not manufactured in the United States, so quality control may be poor.

In mid-2007 the Food and Drug Administration (FDA) released GMP guidelines for dietary supplements. These rules are expected to prevent variations in the amount of any ingredient contained, the inclusion of ingredients not listed on the label, and the presence of contaminants. Large companies that produce supplements will likely have little difficulty complying with the new regulations, but some smaller companies will need to make substantial changes. These new rules will be fully in force by June 2010. For more information about supplement safety, see appendix A.

Muscle-Building Supplements

Various dietary supplements are sold for the purpose of increasing muscle mass. Protein supplements are among the most popular, although the protein they contain is not different from the type of protein found in food. Creatine supplements may indirectly help some strength and power athletes build muscle by allowing them to perform more repetitions when resistance training. Some supplements are touted as legal alternatives to anabolic steroids (for example, dehydroepiandrosterone, known as DHEA), whereas others claim to influence a particular step in the biochemical process of building muscle (for example, beta-hydroxy-beta-methylbutyrate, known as HMB). Their effectiveness, however, has not been proved. Table 9.1 gives an overview of selected muscle-building supplements.

TABLE 9.1

Overview of Muscle-Building Supplements

Product	Safety*	Effectiveness	Advantages	Disadvantages
Protein powder	Considered safe	Considered effective but no more or less effective than food proteins	Portable, convenient	Typically more expensive than nonfat milk or egg whites; may have unpleasant taste or odor
Creatine	Considered safe	Can increase muscle creatine stores by up to 20%, which can lead to more repetitions of high-intensity exercise (for example, resistance or sprint training)	Convenient	Additional water weight may hamper efforts to make weight or affect speed and flexibility; transient benefit
DHEA	Safety concerns about short-term and long-term use	Not effective		May cause hormone-related side effects (for example, breast development in males and facial hair in females)
HMB	Considered safe	Does not appear to be effective in trained athletes		Cost

*In healthy adults; no large-scale studies have been conducted in children or adolescents.

Protein Supplements

Perhaps no nutrient is more closely tied to increasing muscle mass than protein. Not surprisingly, athletes who want to gain weight by increasing lean body mass almost immediately wonder whether protein supplements can help them achieve their goal and achieve it more quickly than food alone. The truth is that protein supplements are neither more nor less effective than food proteins for building muscle mass. In fact, protein supplements are derived from the proteins found in food. The big issue for athletes who use protein supplements is how the supplements fit into their overall diet. Recall that, when calories are adequate, a protein intake greater than 2 grams per kilogram of body weight has no additional benefit for building muscle.

Protein Powders. Protein powder, which is mixed with water or an artificially sweetened beverage, is one of the most popular supplements with strength and power athletes. Many protein powders contain about 25 grams of high-quality protein per serving, which provides approximately 10 grams of the essential amino acids. Research studies have shown that consuming at least 6 grams of essential amino acids along with some carbohydrate within the first hour after resistance exercise stimulates muscle protein synthesis and aids in recovery.

By itself, protein powder does not taste good, so powdered protein supplements usually contain a small amount of fat and carbohydrate to make them more palatable. The nutrient content of protein powders is essentially the same as that contained in many lean protein foods (see table 9.2). The advantage of a protein powder is that it is portable and convenient, but it can be expensive and the taste can be unpleasant. The advantage to lean protein foods is variety, the array of vitamins and minerals that naturally occur in those foods, and the cost, particularly of milk. The disadvantage is convenience because many protein-rich foods have to be refrigerated, prepared, or cooked.

TABLE 9.2

Protein Powder and Lean Protein Foods Comparison

	Energy (kcal)	Protein (g)	Carbohydrate (g)	Fat (g)	Contains at least 6 g essential amino acids
1 scoop (33 g) protein powder	130	25*	1	2	Usually (check label)
~3 oz (85 g) skinless light meat chicken, roasted	130	23	0	3	Yes
6 oz (170 g) light tuna packed in water	150	32.5	0	1	Yes

*Protein content varies slightly depending on the product.

Weight-Gainer Beverages and Protein Bars. Traditional protein powders contain predominantly protein, whereas weight-gainer products contain carbohydrate and fat in addition to protein because an increase in muscle mass requires sufficient calories as well as an adequate amount of protein. These

TABLE 9.3

Comparison of Three Protein-Containing Products

	Energy (kcal)	Protein (g)	Carbohydrate (g)	Fat (g)
1 scoop (34 g) weight-gainer powder in 8 oz (240 ml) water	155	9*	26	2
8 oz (240 ml) low-fat (1%) chocolate milk	158	8	26	3
1 protein bar (78 g)	310	28	30	10

*Protein content typically ranges from 9 to 14 g depending on the product.

products typically have more protein than traditional protein powders, but most of the calories come from carbohydrate that is usually derived from both starches and sugars. As you can see in table 9.3, this type of product is equivalent to low-fat chocolate milk. Both make an excellent recovery beverage if consumed within the first hour after exercise.

The advantages of a weight-gainer powder are convenience, portability, and cost. Athletes can buy the powder in bulk at reasonable cost and transport it easily because it does not need refrigeration. Low-fat chocolate milk is tasty but may need to be refrigerated, unless it is in a shelf-stable container. The costs will vary, but nonfat or chocolate milk is typically the cheapest dairy product. Many protein supplements are beverages, but hundreds of protein and energy bars that have added protein are also available. In the United States, these products are legally considered foods, not supplements, but they are mentioned here because many athletes consider them protein supplements. Most protein bars contain an equal amount of protein and carbohydrate, usually 25 to 30 grams of each, as well as some fat (table 9.3). The protein portion provides the amino acid building blocks, and the carbohydrate and fat supply the energy needed for building tissue. Energy bars typically contain less protein and fewer calories than protein bars do. Compare the nutrient information on the label.

Protein bars are often higher in fat than protein-containing beverages are. That feature is an advantage if the athlete needs the additional calories or needs to satisfy her or his hunger for several hours. The additional calories can be a disadvantage for athletes who are trying to lose or stabilize weight, so a protein-containing food with fewer calories, such as skim milk, may be a better postexercise choice. Protein bars are easy to carry in a workout bag, backpack, or purse but are among the most expensive protein supplement choices, gram for gram.

Whey and Casein. The source of protein in most supplements is typically one of the following: milk protein, whey protein, casein, egg white powder, or soy protein isolate. In the past, egg white was considered the highest quality protein, but a newer, more precise method for determining protein quality has shown that all the protein sources just mentioned are of high quality. Although any of these sources can be used in protein supplements, the most common are whey and casein.

Whey and casein are both milk proteins. When milk is processed, the whey is found in the liquid portion and can be further manufactured into whey protein isolate, whey protein concentrate, or whey powder. Of the three, only whey protein isolate is lactose free. Whey protein isolate is pure protein because both the carbohydrate and fat have been removed. This form is what most athletes buy because it is high in essential amino acids. These amino acids are rapidly absorbed, so whey protein isolate is often advertised as a fast-acting protein. This advantage is important when time is of the essence, such as when consuming amino acids immediately after exercise to stimulate muscle protein synthesis. The price of a protein powder reflects the type of whey that it contains. The most expensive powder has 100 percent whey protein isolate, whereas cheaper powders contain a blend of isolate and concentrate.

Casein is found in the semisolid or curd portion when milk is processed. Casein is often described as a slow-acting protein because it is absorbed much slower than whey protein isolate is. Casein is high in glutamine, a source of energy for immune cells when the body is stressed by endurance exercise or illness.

Several research studies have demonstrated that resistance-trained male athletes who consumed whey protein isolate gained more lean tissue than did those who consumed casein, but other studies have not. Some of these studies have also shown that subjects gained muscle strength. Positive results have influenced some strength athletes, particularly bodybuilders and football players, to supplement with whey protein isolate to increase lean body mass. Other studies, however, have shown that casein is equal to or better than whey protein isolate for increasing muscle mass, so interpreting the results is difficult.

As far as the type of protein that should be taken after exercise, the consensus is that athletes are wise to consume one of the following: a low-fat milk product, a lean animal protein food, or a protein supplement with both whey and casein. The combination of whey and casein, rather than one or the other, is a way to ensure that the body receives both fast- and slow-acting proteins within one hour after exercise.

Creatine

Creatine is one of the most widely studied dietary supplements, so a lot of scientific information is available about its safety and effectiveness in adults. Numerous studies have shown that creatine supplements are safe in healthy adults and that supplementation may increase muscle creatine by 20 percent. This issue is important for strength and power athletes because high-intensity exercise rapidly depletes muscle creatine. The greatest benefits have been seen in athletes who perform repeated sprints or bouts of high-intensity exercise separated by short rest intervals. Creatine supplements may help these athletes train harder (for example, do more repetitions), and the increased training may have a positive effect on performance. Not all athletes, however, respond equally to creatine; performance benefits are not universal.

Weight gain is a reported side effect of creatine supplementation and could be a result of several mechanisms. Increased resistance training (in the presence of a proper diet) is a stimulus for muscle protein synthesis and could be considered an indirect effect of supplementation. Creatine supplementation directly increases the size of muscle cells because of increased intracellular water, which in turn may be a stimulus for increased glycogen storage. Some researchers speculate that the increased cellular water may also stimulate protein synthesis, but more research is needed to advance understanding of the mechanisms. Therefore, a reasonable assumption is that many strength and power athletes will experience an increase in lean body mass (for example, muscle, fluid, and glycogen) with the use of creatine supplements. This increase is likely to persist for several weeks after creatine supplementation ends.

In many cases, the increase in lean body mass would not be detrimental to performance. Extra body weight, however, may reduce speed and flexibility, which would be detrimental to running performance and in sports where the power-to-weight ratio is important. Athletes who must certify weight before competition should be aware that creatine supplementation affects body weight. For many strength and power athletes, the potential benefits of creatine outweigh the potential risks, and those risks appear to be manageable.

Prohormones (DHEA and Androstenedione)

A prohormone is a compound that is a precursor needed to form a hormone. When trying to gain weight as muscle, the focus is testosterone, a hormone manufactured in the body that influences the synthesis of muscle protein. The manufacture of testosterone begins with a cholesterol molecule. Late in the biochemical conversion process two compounds, DHEA and androstenedione (often referred to as andro), are precursors to testosterone. When athletes use the supplement term *prohormones* they are usually referring to these compounds.

Increasing the amount of testosterone in the body to maximum concentration would likely produce an increase in muscle mass. Anabolic steroids are synthetic compounds (drugs) that are nearly identical to testosterone. Unless prescribed by a doctor for the treatment of a medical condition, the use of anabolic steroids, however, is illegal, and most sports governing bodies ban these drugs for ethical and safety reasons. Therefore, athletes are extremely interested in the precursor compounds.

The immediate precursor to testosterone is androstenedione (andro). Androstenedione is illegal to market in the United States because the FDA considers it impure and unsafe. Additionally, the rules of most sports ban it. Essentially, only one prohormone is legally sold as a dietary supplement to athletes—dehydroepiandrosterone (DHEA).

DHEA is naturally secreted by the adrenal glands. It is a precursor, first, to androstenedione synthesis, and, ultimately, to testosterone and estrogen synthesis. Because of its indirect effect on testosterone, DHEA is considered a weak steroid. Athletes who take DHEA supplements often do so in the hope that DHEA will increase testosterone and result in increased protein synthesis of skeletal muscle. This idea sounds good in theory, but does it occur in practice?

Research studies have generally found that DHEA supplementation by young adult athletes does not result in an increase in muscle size or strength. DHEA secretion is normally high in adolescents and young adults, and the amount of testosterone that can be produced naturally has limits. In fact, supplemental DHEA may cause unwanted side effects such as an increase in breast tissue in males (remember that DHEA is also a precursor to estrogen) and growth of facial hair in females. These side effects probably occur because DHEA upsets the hormonal balance of the body. DHEA sounds as if it should work for athletes, but research studies have not shown that it does. The potential benefits are low compared with the potential risks. DHEA supplements are not recommended for children or adolescents.

Beta-Hydroxy-Beta-Methylbutyrate

One of the reasons that athletes take beta-hydroxy-beta-methylbutyrate (HMB) is the hope of increasing muscle size. HMB is a by-product of the metabolism of leucine, an essential amino acid. A 3-gram dose, which is considered safe in adults, is theorized to increase muscle size because of the effect of HMB on reducing the breakdown of muscle cell protein following resistance exercise. The studies that have found an increase in lean body mass with HMB supplementation have most often been conducted in untrained athletes. In trained athletes, HMB supplementation typically does not result in a change in body composition. This result makes sense because the initiation of resistance training is a temporary stress on the body that results in an increase in protein turnover. With chronic resistance training, however, the body makes adaptations that can offset an increase in protein turnover. Thus, in trained athletes who want to change body composition, HMB supplements appear to have low potential risk but also little potential benefit. HMB supplements are not recommended for children or adolescents.

Fat-Loss Supplements

The process of weight loss through diet and exercise is intense and continuous. Adhering to a program requires a high degree of motivation daily. Even under the best circumstances the loss of body fat is challenging, takes a relatively long time, and can leave you feeling less energetic because you are restricting food intake. Not surprisingly, then, some of the most popular supplements on the market are related to quick weight loss. Table 9.4 gives an overview of selected fat-loss supplements.

TABLE 9.4

Overview of Fat-Loss Supplements

Product	Safety*	Effectiveness	Advantages	Disadvantages
Ephedra, ma huang (ephedrine)	Banned in most sports and by some states; banned for sale in the U.S. if dose is greater than 10 mg A likely contributor in a few cases when professional athletes have died in training	Effective as a central nervous system stimulant With caffeine, effective for short term (6 months) 8–9 lb (3.6–4.1 kg) weight loss in obese people		Banned substance Side effects (headache, insomnia, increased blood pressure, increased heart rate) Amount in the supplement can vary Purity is questionable
Citrus aurantium (bitter orange)	Banned by many sports governing bodies Similar safety concerns and side effects as ephedra	Possibly effective for very short-term (2 months or less) 5–7 lb (2.3–3.2 kg) weight loss in overweight or obese people		Banned substance Contains synephrine Amount in the supplement can vary Purity is questionable
Guarana or maté, extracts (herbal source of caffeine)	Probably safe if taken in moderation (less than 300 mg of caffeine daily)	Not effective for weight loss	Taste may be appealing	Rapid heartbeat, nausea, and symptoms associated with withdrawal (headache and fatigue)
Green tea extract (contains caffeine and other compounds)	Probably safe if taken in moderation (less than 300 mg of caffeine daily)	May cause slight elevation in metabolic rate	Taste may be appealing	Side effects (insomnia, rapid heartbeat, nausea) Withdrawal symptoms (headache and fatigue)
Yohimbe extract	Not safe for women, adolescents, children, or those with mental illness Should not be taken with alcohol, diuretics, or medications used to treat depression or high blood pressure	Not effective for changing body composition		High potential for risk Amount in the supplement can vary Purity is questionable
Carnitine	Probably safe at 2–4 g/day	Not effective to increase fatty acid metabolism or for weight loss		Cost
Conjugated linoleic acid (CLA)	Probably safe at 3.2 g/day if properly formulated Some forms may be pro-inflammatory	Effective for extremely slow weight loss (~3 oz or 90 g, per week)	Good source of an essential fatty acid if food sources are not consumed	Cost May promote inflammation

* In healthy adults; not recommended for use by children or adolescents.
Data from Haaz, Fontaine, Cutter et al. 2006; Shekelle, Hardy, Morton et al. 2003; Terpstra 2004; and Whigham, Watras, and Schoeller 2007.

These products are often called fat burners because they increase fat metabolism. Most weight-loss supplements contain at least one active ingredient that stimulates metabolism. When metabolic rate increases, more calories are needed, and if food intake remains the same the increased calories will come from stored body fat. Although many active ingredients may be used to stimulate metabolism, the most popular ones are ephedra, caffeine, and extracts of bitter orange, green tea, and yohimbe. All these products stimulate metabolism, and most slightly depress appetite. The effect on metabolism is typically small. An obese person using any of these products would likely lose less than 10 pounds (4.5 kilograms) over six months. The amount that a nonobese athlete might lose is unknown.

One reason that fat burners are especially popular is that they are also energy boosters. In other words, they contain compounds that stimulate the central nervous system so that the user temporarily feels less fatigued. But these supplements have side effects that are characteristic of stimulants, such as rapid heartbeat and increased blood pressure.

Most stimulants are addictive. Athletes may become dependent on continued intake because the withdrawal symptoms—headache, fatigue, irritability, and inability to concentrate—can negatively affect training, performance, and general well-being. These products may contain active ingredients banned by sports governing bodies or be contaminated with other banned substances. Some may cause a positive drug test. At the very least, athletes should read labels carefully to determine the contents and consider the problems that may be associated with these supplements.

Ephedrine and Caffeine

One of the most controversial weight-loss supplements for athletes is ephedrine, sometimes known as ephedra. Technically, *Ephedra* is a plant genus from which the active ingredient ephedrine may be extracted, but in everyday language ephedrine and ephedra are often used interchangeably. Ma huang is an herbal extract that contains ephedrine. The stimulatory properties of ephedrine have long been known. Medications used to treat asthma and nasal congestion often include ephedrine.

Ephedrine has a narrow dose range, meaning that the difference between a safe dose and an unsafe dose is relatively small. Nearly all ephedrine-containing supplements also contain some form of caffeine because caffeine enhances the effectiveness of ephedrine. No evidence is available that caffeine by itself is an effective weight-loss agent. Studies of obese subjects have shown that ephedrine and caffeine together can produce a weight loss of about 8 to 9 pounds (3.6 to 4.1 kilograms) over a six-month period. None of these studies have been conducted in athletes, and whether this combination would have the same effect in those who are not obese is not known.

The sale of ephedrine-containing supplements in the United States increased in 1994 when laws governing sales of dietary supplements were changed. By 1997 secondhand accounts surfaced that ephedrine was respon-

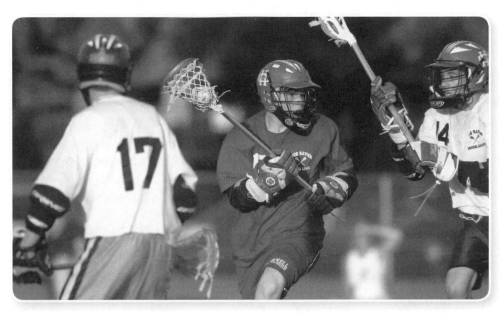

Athletes in many sports, including lacrosse, who wish to reduce their body fat to increase their speed or mobility should carefully weigh the potential risks and benefits of fat-loss supplements.

sible for a handful of deaths to otherwise healthy adults. In 2000 scientific evidence showed that some ephedra supplements were not pure and had markedly more ephedrine than was stated on the label.

In 2001 the high-profile death of a professional football player who was trying to lose weight rapidly while practicing in hot and humid conditions caused the National Football League to ban ephedrine-containing supplements. Many sport governing bodies followed suit, but not Major League Baseball. In 2003 a major league pitching prospect died at spring training in hot and humid conditions after using ephedrine. Following his death, the FDA enacted a ban in 2004 on the sale of all ephedrine-containing dietary supplements across the United States, but a federal court later struck down portions of the ban. At present, low-dose (10 milligrams or less) ephedrine-containing supplements are legal to sell and purchase in the United States, unless a state enacts its own ban, as California and New York have.

Supplements that contain ephedrine present a high potential risk because of concerns about purity, legality, and safety, especially to those who are training or competing in hot and humid environments and are trying to lose weight rapidly. For these reasons, ephedrine-containing supplements are not recommended.

Citrus Aurantium *(Bitter Orange)*

Following the FDA ban, many ephedra-containing dietary supplements were reformulated to be ephedrine free. Synephrine or related compounds can replace ephedrine because they have similar biochemical properties. These compounds are often extracted from the plant *Citrus aurantium*, also known as bitter orange. Bitter orange extract has now become one of the top five ingredients in weight-loss products sold in the United States, and its sales volume may eventually surpass the sales volume of ephedra-containing weight-loss supplements.

A small number of studies of less than 100 overweight and obese people have shown some benefit to using dietary supplements with synephrine-related compounds in conjunction with other weight-loss strategies such as reduced caloric intake or increased exercise. On average, the overweight person could expect to lose 2.4 to 3.4 kilograms (about 5 to 7 pounds) of body weight in the short term (two months or less). Many of the safety concerns about synephrine parallel the concerns about ephedrine, specifically the dose that is considered safe. Bitter orange is banned by many sports governing bodies including the NCAA and the NFL. Until more evidence to the contrary appears, the use of bitter orange extract must be considered to have low potential benefit as an effective weight-loss agent for athletes and high potential risk because of concerns about purity and safety. Its use is not recommended.

Guarana, Maté, and Green Tea Extracts

Guarana, maté, and green tea extracts are all sources of caffeine. Guarana seeds contain about four times more caffeine than coffee beans do, and those who are sensitive to the effects of caffeine generally do not tolerate guarana well. Yerba maté seeds also contain caffeine but in relatively low amounts. A tealike drink called maté is typically lower in caffeine than both coffee and black tea. Similarly, green tea extract beverages also contain caffeine but in lower amounts than coffee. Besides caffeine, other active ingredients are present in green tea, and together they may act to produce a slight, temporary increase in metabolic rate.

Studies of guarana and maté use by obese subjects generally find that their effect on weight loss is small or nonexistent, which is not surprising because caffeine is not an effective weight-loss agent. Of the three substances, the most promising is green tea extract because it contains a large number of active ingredients besides caffeine. The interaction of these ingredients may increase metabolism slightly.

These products have low potential benefit and some potential for risk because of caffeine content. A guideline for athletes is that caffeine intake from all sources—beverages, supplements, foods, and medications—should total 300 milligrams or less daily. Eight ounces (240 ml) of brewed coffee contains about 80 to 135 milligrams of caffeine. Caffeine tablets, fat-burning supplements, and herbal teas for weight loss usually contain 200 to 250 milligrams per serving.

Consuming more than 300 milligrams of caffeine daily can adversely affect hydration status because caffeine is a mild diuretic. Intake above this level is considered dangerous for athletes who are cutting weight because high levels of caffeine add to water weight loss and temporarily increase heart rate

The Risk of Multiple Active Ingredients

One of the concerns about dietary supplements sold for weight loss is that they contain multiple active ingredients. An active ingredient is the chemically active part of a substance that causes a reaction or change. In a study of more than 400 products, the average number of ingredients in weight-loss supplements was 10. Consumers are not likely to know the amount (that is, dose) of each ingredient or be able to judge the safety and effectiveness of the product.

Many athletes use these multiple-ingredient weight-loss products when they are cutting weight rapidly because the stimulants in the products mask fatigue and because many of the ingredients are mild diuretics. Serious consequences can occur because the athlete who is cutting weight is already dehydrated, and side effects such as increased heart rate and blood pressure can contribute to life-threatening medical conditions. The narrow safe-dose range of these products narrows even more when the athlete is dehydrated.

and blood pressure at a time of elevated physiologic stress. Intake above 500 milligrams daily is usually associated with unpleasant symptoms such as anxiety, insomnia, gastrointestinal upset, and rapid heartbeat. Some sports governing bodies list caffeine as a banned substance at a certain level, but the amount is so high that athletes would most likely be unable to perform because of the side effects (for example, shaking and rapid heartbeat) of such a high caffeine dose.

Yohimbe Extract

Yohimbe is a tree native to Africa whose bark contains the chemical compound yohimbine. Yohimbine is sold as an herbal dietary supplement, but because it is an extract, the amount found in a yohimbe supplement can vary. Yohimbine is advertised as a way to change body composition (both to reduce fat and to increase muscle mass), but studies have not shown that a benefit exists.

Women, adolescents, children, and those with mental illness should not take yohimbine, nor should it be consumed with alcohol or diuretics. Yohimbine interacts with several medications including those used to treat depression and high blood pressure. For those reasons, yohimbine use by athletes has high potential for risk and little potential benefit. Its use is not recommended.

Carnitine

Carnitine is one of many dietary supplements sold for weight loss that contain compounds that are part of the complicated biochemical pathways that oxidize (burn) fat. Most of these supplements are advertised as a way to burn more fatty acids or burn fatty acids more rapidly. The source of the fatty acids would be stored body fat (adipose tissue). Such supplements are appealing because the user would be taking a pill that would slowly melt away fat. If something sounds too good to be true, it probably is. Many of these supplements are simply too good to be true.

Carnitine is necessary to transport fatty acids across the inner membrane of cell mitochondria, where the fat will eventually be burned for energy. Carnitine is found in food, and the body can manufacture it, so humans are unlikely to be deficient. Taking a large amount of carnitine as a supplement is unlikely to have a substantial effect on fatty acid metabolism because the transport of carnitine into cells is well controlled.

The effect of carnitine supplements on weight loss would be indirect. An increase in carnitine is theorized to increase the rate of fat oxidization (burning), which would result in a loss of body fat. Studies have not supported this theory. Most studies have used a dose of 2 to 4 grams per day, a dosage that appears to be safe. For the purpose of weight (fat) loss, carnitine supplements appear to have low potential risk and extremely low potential benefit.

Conjugated Linoleic Acid

Conjugated linoleic acid is one of a handful of naturally occurring compounds in the body that influence the deposition of fatty acids into adipose tissue (body fat). Linoleic acid is a fatty acid that the body cannot manufacture. Conjugated linoleic acid (CLA) is mixture of linoleic acid molecules, each with a slightly different chemical structure (that is, isomer). CLA occurs naturally in meat and dairy foods. CLA supplements have a different isomer mixture, including the isomer trans-10, cis-12, than that found in food and have been shown to decrease body fat in animals. This supplement has always held great promise because studies in mice demonstrated a significant increase in fat loss resulting from the effects of CLA on two enzymes associated with storing fat in adipose tissue.

On the basis of at least 18 studies, some of which were conducted in normal-weight or overweight people who were engaged in resistance training, those who consumed CLA supplements lost approximately .09 kilogram (0.2 pound) per week compared with those who received a placebo. This amount of weight loss is small but statistically significant. To put it in perspective, the average American gains 0.009 kilogram (0.02 pound) per week.

Concerns have arisen about safety of CLA supplements because some studies have shown that CLA is proinflammatory. Inflammation is the response of the body to injury, invasion, or disease, triggering a sequence of immune reactions. At the cellular level, inflammation increases the risk of heart disease. A dose of 3.2 grams of CLA per day is considered safe and effective, but the CLA supplement should contain an equal mix of just two isomers (cis-9, trans-11 and trans-10, cis-12), because research studies suggest that these forms are most beneficial. Unfortunately, manufacturers are not required to list the specific isomer information on the label.

PART III

Meal Plans
for Making Weight

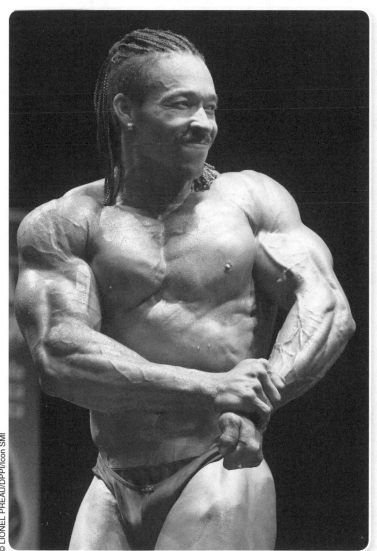

© LIONEL PREAU/DPPI/Icon SMI

Building Muscle

This chapter is designed for athletes who want to gain muscle mass. (If your goal is to lose body fat, turn to chapter 11. If you want to build muscle *and* lose fat, see chapter 12.) Athletes likely to have this goal include lean athletes who want to increase body weight, size, and muscle to match up better with opponents as well as distance runners and gymnasts who have a low percentage of body fat. With this action plan, your weight will increase because the additional muscle mass will add to total body weight.

To be successful in meeting your goal of increasing muscle mass, you must do three things:

- Consume the right number of calories
- Consume the proper amounts and proportions of protein, carbohydrate, and fat
- Engage in a program of resistance exercise

To determine the number of calories that you should consume while building muscle, you need to determine your baseline calorie intake. If your current body weight is stable, you can use the figures that you obtained in calculating your average daily caloric intake as explained in chapter 3. Thus, your current intake becomes your baseline. You should also calculate your estimated caloric needs as explained in chapter 5. Because you are not trying to lose weight, your current intake should be close to your estimated caloric needs. If your current intake is less than your caloric needs, you may be undereating. A large discrepancy between your current intake and your estimated caloric needs may hamper your efforts to gain muscle mass. Calories are key! You must take in enough calories to support resistance training and fuel muscle growth.

When you determine your baseline calorie intake, factor in a calorie increase as shown in table 10.1. To gain muscle mass, males should add 400 to 500 kilocalories daily to their baseline estimate. The recommendation for females is to add 300 to 400 kilocalories daily to the baseline number. A range is given because the number of calories needed cannot be predicted exactly. A good guideline is to start at the lower end of the range. Estimating your actual energy needs is problematic. For that reason, you should evaluate your progress regularly to assess whether you are within an appropriate calorie range and be ready to adjust as needed.

TABLE 10.1

Calories Needed to Gain Muscle

Goal	Gender	Total calories
To gain muscle mass	Male	Baseline kcal plus 400 to 500 kcal
	Female	Baseline kcal plus 300 to 400 kcal

Select Your Jumpstart Meal Plan

After you know how many calories you need, you are ready to choose a jumpstart meal plan for that calorie level. The plans in this chapter are simple and are intended to give you a jumpstart on your effort to build muscle. You should use these plans only temporarily to help you get started on achieving your goal. The plans offer a limited number of food choices so they are easy to follow. By following these plans exactly, you can establish a pattern of eating that will help you reach your body-composition and performance goals.

Although the simplicity of the plans makes getting started on your goal easy, it also results in a lack of variety. A monotonous diet is difficult to follow over time, so do not use this plan for more than a week or two. After that, you can use the precision meal planning system in chapter 13 to create a customized personal plan that will expand the variety of foods. By creating a diet with your favorite foods and with a greater variety of foods, you will be able to follow your plan over the length of time needed to meet your goals.

Each meal plan has been designed to contain the proper amount and proportions of carbohydrate, protein, and fat to support maximum muscle gain. Each contains approximately 8 grams of carbohydrate, 1.8 grams of protein, and between 1 and 2 grams of fat per kilogram of body weight.

Each jumpstart meal plan consists of seven food groups and lists the total number of choices that you need to make from each group. You are free to choose whichever foods you like within each food group. To maintain the correct calorie level and macronutrient balance, you need to eat foods and beverages in the quantities specified in your meal plan.

Find your plan with the following easy steps:

1. Select the correct calorie range for your needs based on table 10.1. The meal plans are provided in 500 kilocalorie increments. For example, if you need 2,700 kilocalories daily, you should look at the 2,600 to 3,000 kilocalories meal plan.

2. According to your calorie level, choose the right number of foods from each food group. For example, a 2,700-kilocalorie diet consists of two choices from the fat-free milk and yogurt group, six choices from the nonstarchy vegetables group, and so on. When you need to select more than one food from a group, you may select any combination of the choices to reach the total number. You may choose each food listed more than once. For example, two fat-free milk and yogurt choices could be two 8-ounce (240-milliliter) glasses of fat-free milk or one 8-ounce (240-milliliter) glass of soy milk and 6 ounces (180 grams) of fat-free yogurt. You have several options in each food group but remember that your total number of choices for the day should not exceed the recommendation for your calorie level.

3. From the foods you choose, create three meals and two snacks. Eat the snacks before and after you exercise.

Five sample menus (each for a different calorie level) have been created to illustrate how to translate your choices from the meal plan into meals and snacks. (See chapter 13 for additional information about how to create meals and snacks.) The meals and snacks that you create may look different from these sample menus because each food group has several foods to choose from. When you divide the total choices in your meal plan into meals and snacks, keep in mind that you should have at least three meals and two snacks each day. To build muscle, you should have some carbohydrate and protein in the first hour after exercise (see chapter 6).

2,600- to 3,000-Calorie Meal Plan

Food group	Food group choices	Calorie level and number of choices
Fat-free milk and yogurt	8 oz (240 ml) fat-free or 1% milk 8 oz (240 ml) soy milk 8 oz (240 ml) low-fat kefir 6 oz (180 g) fat-free yogurt	2,600 kcal: choose 2 2,700 kcal: choose 2 2,800 kcal: choose 2 2,900 kcal: choose 2 3,000 kcal: choose 3
Nonstarchy vegetables	1 cup (56 g) dark green lettuce 15 raw baby carrots 1 large tomato 1/2 cup (62 g) cooked green beans 1/2 cup (78 g) cooked broccoli 1/2 cup (62 g) cooked cauliflower 1/2 cup (90 g) cooked zucchini 1 medium onion 1 bell pepper	2,600 kcal: choose 5 2,700 kcal: choose 6 2,800 kcal: choose 6 2,900 kcal: choose 7 3,000 kcal: choose 6
Fruits	1 small apple 1 small banana 1 cup (144 g) berries 1 small orange 2 tbsp (18 g) raisins 1/2 cup (120 ml) 100% fruit juice 17 grapes 1/2 cup (122 g) unsweetened applesauce 1/2 cup (128 g) cut fresh or canned fruit, unsweetened	2,600 kcal: choose 10 2,700 kcal: choose 10 2,800 kcal: choose 11 2,900 kcal: choose 12 3,000 kcal: choose 12
Grains and starches	1 slice bread 1/2 6-in. (15 cm) pita 1/2 English muffin 1/2 small (2 oz or 60 g) bagel 1/4 large (4 oz or 120 g) bagel 1/2 cup (121 g) cooked cereal 3/4 cup (21 g) unsweetened ready-to-eat cereal 1 4-in. (10 cm) thin pancake 1 4-in. (10 cm) square waffle 1/2 cup (93 g) cooked rice 1/2 cup (70 g) cooked pasta 1/3 cup (83 g) baked beans 1/2 cup (82 g) corn 1/4 large (3 oz or 90 g) cooked potato 1 small dinner roll 3 graham cracker squares	2,600 kcal: choose 10 2,700 kcal: choose 10 2,800 kcal: choose 10 2,900 kcal: choose 10 3,000 kcal: choose 11
Foods with sugar	1 energy or granola bar (~1 oz or 30 g) 1 frozen 100% fruit juice bar 1 tbsp (21 g) honey, jam, or syrup or 1 tbsp (12 g) sugar 1 cup (8 oz or 240 ml) sports drink 1/2 cup (87 g) frozen yogurt	2,600 kcal: choose 4 2,700 kcal: choose 4 2,800 kcal: choose 4 2,900 kcal: choose 4 3,000 kcal: choose 4

Lean protein	1 oz (30 g) (very thin slice) *lean*
	   chicken
	   turkey
	   beef
	   pork
	   fish
	2 egg whites or 1/4 cup (61 g) egg substitute
		2,600 kcal: choose 5
		2,700 kcal: choose 5
		2,800 kcal: choose 6
		2,900 kcal: choose 6
		3,000 kcal: choose 6

Fats and oils	1 tsp (5 g) margarine 1 tbsp (15 g) reduced-fat margarine 1 tsp (5 g) oil 1 tsp (5 g) mayo 1 tbsp (14 g) reduced-fat mayo 1/2 tbsp (8 g) peanut or almond butter 1 tbsp (14 g) cream cheese 1 tbsp (16 g) salad dressing 2 tbsp (29 g) avocado 6 almonds 4 walnut halves 10 peanuts	2,600 kcal: choose 10 2,700 kcal: choose 12 2,800 kcal: choose 12 2,900 kcal: choose 12 3,000 kcal: choose 11

Sample 2,600-Calorie One-Day Menu

Meal or snack	Amount and food	Number of choices and food group
Breakfast	1 1/2 cup (363 g) cooked oatmeal	3 grains and starches
	2 tbsp (18 g) raisins	1 fruits
	1 tbsp (12 g) sugar	1 foods with sugar
	6 almonds	1 fats and oils
	4 oz (120 ml) orange juice	1 fruits
	8 oz (240 ml) skim milk	1 fat-free milk and yogurt
Lunch	2 slices whole-wheat bread	2 grains and starches
	2 slices (2 oz or 60 g) turkey breast	2 lean protein
	Lettuce and tomato slices	1 nonstarchy vegetable
	2 tsp (10 g) mayo	2 fats and oils
	2 tbsp (29 g) avocado	1 fats and oils
	15 raw baby carrots	1 nonstarchy vegetable
	34 grapes	2 fruits
	Calorie-free beverage	
Preexercise snack	1 large banana	2 fruits
	8 oz (1 cup or 240 ml) sports drink	1 foods with sugar
Postexercise snack	6 oz (180 g) fat-free yogurt	1 fat-free milk and yogurt
	1 medium-large apple	2 fruits
	1 tbsp (16 g) peanut butter	2 fats and oils
	16 oz (2 cups or 480 ml) sports drink	2 foods with sugar
Dinner	3 oz (90g) baked, skinless chicken breast	3 lean protein
	1/2 cup (82 g) corn	1 grains and starches
	2/3 cup (166 g) baked beans	2 grains and starches
	1 cup (56 g) dark green lettuce	1 nonstarchy vegetable
	1 bell pepper	1 nonstarchy vegetable
	1 large tomato	1 nonstarchy vegetable
	2 tbsp (32 g) salad dressing	2 fats and oils
	2 whole-grain rolls	2 grains and starches
	2 tsp (10 g) margarine	2 fats and oils
	1 cup (244 g) unsweetened applesauce	2 fruits

3,100- to 3,500-Calorie Meal Plan

Food group	Food group choices	Calorie level and number of choices
Fat-free milk and yogurt	8 oz (240 ml) fat-free or 1% milk 8 oz (240 ml) soy milk 8 oz (240 ml) low-fat kefir 6 oz (180 g) fat-free yogurt	3,100 kcal: choose 3 3,200 kcal: choose 3 3,300 kcal: choose 3 3,400 kcal: choose 3 3,500 kcal: choose 3
Nonstarchy vegetables	1 cup (56 g) dark green lettuce 15 raw baby carrots 1 large tomato 1/2 cup (62 g) cooked green beans 1/2 cup (78 g) cooked broccoli 1/2 cup (62 g) cooked cauliflower 1/2 cup (90 g) cooked zucchini 1 medium onion 1 bell pepper	3,100 kcal: choose 6 3,200 kcal: choose 6 3,300 kcal: choose 6 3,400 kcal: choose 6 3,500 kcal: choose 6
Fruits	1 small apple 1 small banana 1 cup (144 g) berries 1 small orange 2 tbsp (18 g) raisins 1/2 cup (120 ml) 100% fruit juice 17 grapes 1/2 cup (122 g) unsweetened applesauce 1/2 cup (128 g) cut fresh or canned fruit, unsweetened	3,100 kcal: choose 12 3,200 kcal: choose 12 3,300 kcal: choose 12 3,400 kcal: choose 13 3,500 kcal: choose 13
Grains and starches	1 slice bread 1/2 6-in. (15 cm) pita 1/2 English muffin 1/2 small (2 oz or 60 g) bagel 1/4 large (4 oz or 120 g) bagel 1/2 cup (121 g) cooked cereal 3/4 cup (21 g) unsweetened ready-to-eat cereal 1 4-in. (10 cm) thin pancake 1 4-in. (10 cm) square waffle 1/2 cup (93 g) cooked rice 1/2 cup (70 g) cooked pasta 1/3 cup (83 g) baked beans 1/2 cup (82 g) corn 1/4 large (3 oz or 90 g) potato 1 small dinner roll 3 graham cracker squares	3,100 kcal: choose 11 3,200 kcal: choose 13 3,300 kcal: choose 13 3,400 kcal: choose 14 3,500 kcal: choose 13
Foods with sugar	1 energy or granola bar (~1 oz or 30 g) 1 frozen 100% fruit juice bar 1 tbsp (21 g) honey, jam, or syrup or 1 tbsp (12 g) sugar 1 cup (8 oz or 240 ml) sports drink 1/2 cup (87 g) frozen yogurt	3,100 kcal: choose 4 3,200 kcal: choose 4 3,300 kcal: choose 5 3,400 kcal: choose 5 3,500 kcal: choose 5

Lean protein	1 oz (30 g) (very thin slice) *lean*
	   chicken
	   turkey
	   beef
	   pork
	   fish
	2 egg whites or 1/4 cup (61 g) egg substitute
		3,100 kcal: choose 6
		3,200 kcal: choose 7
		3,300 kcal: choose 7
		3,400 kcal: choose 7
		3,500 kcal: choose 7

Fats and oils	1 tsp (5 g) margarine 1 tbsp (15 g) reduced-fat margarine 1 tsp (5 g) oil 1 tsp (5 g) mayo 1 tbsp (14 g) reduced-fat mayo 1/2 tbsp (8 g) peanut or almond butter 1 tbsp (14 g) cream cheese 1 tbsp (16 g) salad dressing 2 tbsp (29 g) avocado 6 almonds 4 walnut halves 10 peanuts	3,100 kcal: choose 14 3,200 kcal: choose 11 3,300 kcal: choose 12 3,400 kcal: choose 12 3,500 kcal: choose 15

3,600- to 4,000-Calorie Meal Plan

Food group	Food group choices	Calorie level and number of choices
Fat-free milk and yogurt	8 oz (240 ml) fat-free or 1% milk 8 oz (240 ml) soy milk 8 oz (240 ml) low-fat kefir 6 oz (180 g) fat-free yogurt	3,600 kcal: choose 3 3,700 kcal: choose 3 3,800 kcal: choose 3 3,900 kcal: choose 3 4,000 kcal: choose 3
Nonstarchy vegetables	1 cup (56 g) dark green lettuce 15 raw baby carrots 1 large tomato 1/2 cup (62 g) cooked green beans 1/2 cup (78 g) cooked broccoli 1/2 cup (62 g) cooked cauliflower 1/2 cup (90 g) cooked zucchini 1 medium onion 1 bell pepper	3,600 kcal: choose 5 3,700 kcal: choose 5 3,800 kcal: choose 5 3,900 kcal: choose 5 4,000 kcal: choose 6
Fruits	1 small apple 1 small banana 1 cup (144 g) berries 1 small orange 2 tbsp (18 g) raisins 1/2 cup (120 ml) 100% fruit juice 17 grapes 1/2 cup (122 g) unsweetened applesauce 1/2 cup (128 g) cut fresh or canned fruit, unsweetened	3,600 kcal: choose 12 3,700 kcal: choose 12 3,800 kcal: choose 12 3,900 kcal: choose 13 4,000 kcal: choose 13
Grains and starches	1 slice bread 1/2 6-in. (15 cm) pita 1/2 English muffin 1/2 small (2 oz or 60 g) bagel 1/4 large (4 oz or 120 g) bagel 1/2 cup (121 g) cooked cereal 3/4 cup (21 g) unsweetened ready-to-eat cereal 1 4-in. (10 cm) thin pancake 1 4-in. (10 cm) square waffle 1/2 cup (93 g) cooked rice 1/2 cup (70 g) cooked pasta 1/3 cup (83 g) baked beans 1/2 cup 82 g) corn 1/4 large (3 oz or 90 g) potato 1 small dinner roll 3 graham cracker squares	3,600 kcal: choose 12 3,700 kcal: choose 13 3,800 kcal: choose 14 3,900 kcal: choose 15 4,000 kcal: choose 16
Foods with sugar	1 energy or granola bar (~1 oz or 30 g) 1 frozen 100% fruit juice bar 1 tbsp (21 g) honey, jam, or syrup or 1 tbsp (12 g) sugar 1 cup (8 oz or 240 ml) sports drink 1/2 cup (87 g) frozen yogurt	3,600 kcal: choose 5 3,700 kcal: choose 5 3,800 kcal: choose 5 3,900 kcal: choose 5 4,000 kcal: choose 5

Lean protein	1 oz (30 g) (very thin slice) *lean*
	   chicken
	   turkey
	   beef
	   pork
	   fish
	2 egg whites or 1/4 cup (61 g) egg substitute
		3,600 kcal: choose 8
		3,700 kcal: choose 8
		3,800 kcal: choose 8
		3,900 kcal: choose 8
		4,000 kcal: choose 8

Fats and oils	1 tsp (5 g) margarine 1 tbsp (15 g) reduced-fat margarine 1 tsp (5 g) oil 1 tsp (5 g) mayo 1 tbsp (14 g) reduced-fat mayo 1/2 tbsp (8 g) peanut or almond butter 1 tbsp (14 g) cream cheese 1 tbsp (16 g) salad dressing 2 tbsp (29 g) avocado 6 almonds 4 walnut halves 10 peanuts	3,600 kcal: choose 19 3,700 kcal: choose 20 3,800 kcal: choose 20 3,900 kcal: choose 20 4,000 kcal: choose 20

Sample 3,600-Calorie One-Day Menu

Meal or snack	Amount and food	Number of choices and food group
Breakfast	1 1/2 cup (363 g) cooked oatmeal	3 grains and starches
	2 tbsp (18 g) raisins	1 fruits
	1 tbsp (12 g) sugar	1 foods with sugar
	2 tsp (10 g) margarine	2 fats and oils
	12 almonds	2 fats and oils
	8 oz (240 ml) orange juice	2 fruits
	8 oz (240 ml) skim milk	1 fat-free milk and yogurt
Lunch	2 slices whole-wheat bread	2 grains and starches
	3 slices (3 oz or 90 g) turkey breast	3 lean protein
	1 tbsp (15 g) mayo	3 fats and oils
	4 tbsp (58 g) avocado	2 fats and oils
	Lettuce and tomato slices	1 nonstarchy vegetable
	15 raw baby carrots	1 nonstarchy vegetable
	1/3 cup (83 g) baked beans	1 grains and starches
	34 grapes	2 fruits
	Calorie-free beverage	
Preexercise snack	1 large banana	2 fruits
	6 graham cracker squares	2 grains and starches
	16 oz (2 cups or 480 ml) sports drink	2 foods with sugar
Postexercise snack	6 oz (180 g) fat-free yogurt	1 fat-free milk and yogurt
	1/2 cup (128 g) canned peaches, unsweetened	1 fruits
	1 medium-large apple	2 fruits
	2 tbsp (32 g) peanut butter	4 fats and oils
	16 oz (2 cups or 480 ml) sports drink	2 foods with sugar
Dinner	5 oz (150 g) baked, skinless chicken breast	5 lean protein
	1/2 cup (82 g) corn	1 grains and starches
	2/3 cup (166 g) baked beans	2 grains and starches
	1 cup (56 g) dark green lettuce	1 nonstarchy vegetable
	1 bell pepper	1 nonstarchy vegetable
	1 large tomato	1 nonstarchy vegetable
	2 tbsp (32 g) salad dressing	2 fats and oils
	1 whole-grain roll	1 grains and starches
	4 tsp (20 g) margarine	4 fats and oils
	1 cup (244 g) unsweetened applesauce	2 fruits
	8 oz (240 ml) skim milk	1 fat-free milk and yogurt

4,100- to 4,500-Calorie Meal Plan

Food group	Food group choices	Calorie level and number of choices
Fat-free milk and yogurt	8 oz (240 ml) fat-free or 1% milk 8 oz (240 ml) soy milk 8 oz (240 ml) low-fat kefir 6 oz (180 g) fat-free yogurt	4,100 kcal: choose 3 4,200 kcal: choose 3 4,300 kcal: choose 3 4,400 kcal: choose 3 4,500 kcal: choose 3
Nonstarchy vegetables	1 cup (56 g) dark green lettuce 15 raw baby carrots 1 large tomato 1/2 cup (62 g) cooked green beans 1/2 cup (78 g) cooked broccoli 1/2 cup (62 g) cooked cauliflower 1/2 cup (90 g) cooked zucchini 1 medium onion 1 bell pepper	4,100 kcal: choose 6 4,200 kcal: choose 6 4,300 kcal: choose 6 4,400 kcal: choose 6 4,500 kcal: choose 6
Fruits	1 small apple 1 small banana 1 cup (144 g) berries 1 small orange 2 tbsp (18 g) raisins 1/2 cup (120 ml) 100% fruit juice 17 grapes 1/2 cup (122 g) unsweetened applesauce 1/2 cup (128 g) cut fresh or canned fruit, unsweetened	4,100 kcal: choose 13 4,200 kcal: choose 13 4,300 kcal: choose 13 4,400 kcal: choose 14 4,500 kcal: choose 14
Grains and starches	1 slice bread 1/2 6-in. (15 cm) pita 1/2 English muffin 1/2 small (2 oz or 60 g) bagel 1/4 large (4 oz or 120 g)bagel 1/2 cup (121 g) cooked cereal 3/4 cup (21 g) unsweetened ready-to-eat cereal 1 4-in. (10 cm) thin pancake 1 4-in. (10 cm) square waffle 1/2 cup (93 g) cooked rice 1/2 cup (70 g) cooked pasta 1/3 cup (83 g) baked beans 1/2 cup (82 g) corn 1/4 large (3 oz or 90 g) potato 1 small dinner roll 3 graham cracker squares	4,100 kcal: choose 16 4,200 kcal: choose 16 4,300 kcal: choose 16 4,400 kcal: choose 16 4,500 kcal: choose 17
Foods with sugar	1 energy or granola bar (~1 oz or 30 g) 1 frozen 100% fruit juice bar 1 tbsp (21 g) honey, jam, or syrup or 1 tbsp (12 g) sugar 1 cup (8 oz or 240 ml) sports drink 1/2 cup (87 g) frozen yogurt	4,100 kcal: choose 6 4,200 kcal: choose 7 4,300 kcal: choose 8 4,400 kcal: choose 8 4,500 kcal: choose 8
Lean protein	1 oz (30 g) (very thin slice) *lean* chicken turkey beef pork fish 2 egg whites or 1/4 cup (61 g) egg substitute	4,100 kcal: choose 8 4,200 kcal: choose 9 4,300 kcal: choose 9 4,400 kcal: choose 10 4,500 kcal: choose 10
Fats and oils	1 tsp (5 g) margarine 1 tbsp (15 g) reduced-fat margarine 1 tsp (5 g) oil 1 tsp (5 g) mayo 1 tbsp (14 g) reduced-fat mayo 1/2 tbsp (8 g) peanut or almond butter 1 tbsp (14 g) cream cheese 1 tbsp (16 g) salad dressing 2 tbsp (29 g) avocado 6 almonds 4 walnut halves 10 peanuts	4,100 kcal: choose 21 4,200 kcal: choose 21 4,300 kcal: choose 21 4,400 kcal: choose 21 4,500 kcal: choose 22

4,600- to 5,000-Calorie Meal Plan

Food group	Food group choices	Calorie level and number of choices
Fat-free milk and yogurt	8 oz (240 ml) fat-free or 1% milk 8 oz (240 ml) soy milk 8 oz (240 ml) low-fat kefir 6 oz (180 g) fat-free yogurt	4,600 kcal: choose 3 4,700 kcal: choose 3 4,800 kcal: choose 4 4,900 kcal: choose 4 5,000 kcal: choose 4
Nonstarchy vegetables	1 cup (56 g) dark green lettuce 15 raw baby carrots 1 large tomato 1/2 cup (62 g) cooked green beans 1/2 cup (78 g) cooked broccoli 1/2 cup (62 g) cooked cauliflower 1/2 cup (90 g) cooked zucchini 1 medium onion 1 bell pepper	4,600 kcal: choose 6 4,700 kcal: choose 6 4,800 kcal: choose 6 4,900 kcal: choose 6 5,000 kcal: choose 6
Fruits	1 small apple 1 small banana 1 cup (144 g) berries 1 small orange 2 tbsp (18 g) raisins 1/2 cup (120 ml) 100% fruit juice 17 grapes 1/2 cup (122 g) unsweetened applesauce 1/2 cup (128 g) cut fresh or canned fruit, unsweetened	4,600 kcal: choose 14 4,700 kcal: choose 14 4,800 kcal: choose 14 4,900 kcal: choose 14 5,000 kcal: choose 15
Grains and starches	1 slice bread 1/2 6-in. (15 cm) pita 1/2 English muffin 1/2 small (2 oz or 60 g) bagel 1/4 large (4 oz or 120 g) bagel 1/2 cup (121 g) cooked cereal 3/4 cup (21 g) unsweetened ready-to-eat cereal 1 4-in. (10 cm) thin pancake 1 4-in. (10 cm) square waffle 1/2 cup (93 g) cooked rice 1/2 cup (70 g) cooked pasta 1/3 cup (83 g) baked beans 1/2 cup (82 g) corn 1/4 large (3 oz or 90 g) potato 1 small dinner roll 3 graham cracker squares	4,600 kcal: choose 18 4,700 kcal: choose 19 4,800 kcal: choose 19 4,900 kcal: choose 19 5,000 kcal: choose 20
Foods with sugar	1 energy or granola bar (~1 oz or 30 g) 1 frozen 100% fruit juice bar 1 tbsp (21 g) honey, jam, or syrup or 1 tbsp (12 g) sugar 1 cup (8 oz or 240 ml) sports drink 1/2 cup (87 g) frozen yogurt	4,600 kcal: choose 8 4,700 kcal: choose 8 4,800 kcal: choose 8 4,900 kcal: choose 9 5,000 kcal: choose 9
Lean protein	1 oz (30 g) (very thin slice) *lean* 　chicken 　turkey 　beef 　pork 　fish 2 egg whites or 1/4 cup (61 g) egg substitute	4,600 kcal: choose 10 4,700 kcal: choose 10 4,800 kcal: choose 10 4,900 kcal: choose 10 5,000 kcal: choose 10
Fats and oils	1 tsp (5 g) margarine 1 tbsp (15 g) reduced-fat margarine 1 tsp (5 g) oil 1 tsp (5 g) mayo 1 tbsp (14 g) reduced-fat mayo 1/2 tbsp (8 g) peanut or almond butter 1 tbsp (14 g) cream cheese 1 tbsp (16 g) salad dressing 2 tbsp (29 g) avocado 6 almonds 4 walnut halves 10 peanuts	4,600 kcal: choose 22 4,700 kcal: choose 23 4,800 kcal: choose 24 4,900 kcal: choose 24 5,000 kcal: choose 24

Sample 4,600-Calorie One-Day Menu

Meal or snack	Amount and food	Number of choices and food group
Breakfast	2 cups (484 g) cooked oatmeal	4 grains and starches
	4 tbsp (36 g) raisins	2 fruits
	2 tbsp (24 g) sugar	2 foods with sugar
	2 tsp (10 g) margarine	2 fats and oils
	18 almonds	3 fats and oils
	8 oz (240 ml) orange juice	2 fruits
	8 oz (240 ml) skim milk	1 fat-free milk and yogurt
Lunch	4 slices whole-wheat bread	4 grains and starches
	4 slices (4 oz or 120 g) turkey breast	4 lean protein
	2 tsp (10 g) mayo	2 fats and oils
	4 tbsp (58 g) avocado	2 fats and oils
	Lettuce and tomato slices	1 nonstarchy vegetable
	15 raw baby carrots	1 nonstarchy vegetable
	34 grapes	2 fruits
	1/2 cup (8 oz or 240 ml) 100% fruit juice	1 fruits
Preexercise snack	1 large banana	2 fruits
	6 graham cracker squares	2 grains and starches
	16 oz (2 cups or 480 ml) sports drink	2 foods with sugar
Postexercise snack	6 oz (180 g) fat-free yogurt	1 fat-free milk and yogurt
	1 small apple	1 fruits
	8 oz (240 ml) 100% fruit juice	2 fruits
	1 small (2 oz or 60 g) bagel	2 grains and starches
	1 1/2 tbsp peanut butter (24 g)	3 fats and oils
	24 oz (720 ml) sports drink	3 foods with sugar
Dinner	6 oz (180 g) baked, skinless chicken breast	6 lean protein
	1 cup (164 g) corn	2 grains and starches
	2/3 cup (166 g) baked beans	2 grains and starches
	2 cups (112 g) dark green lettuce	2 nonstarchy vegetable
	1 bell pepper	1 nonstarchy vegetable
	1 large tomato	1 nonstarchy vegetable
	3 tbsp (48 g) salad dressing	3 fats and oils
	8 walnut halves	2 fats and oils
	2 whole-grain rolls	2 grains and starches
	5 tsp (25 g) margarine	5 fats and oils
	1 tbsp (21 g) honey	1 foods with sugar
	1 cup (244 g) unsweetened applesauce	2 fruits
	8 oz (240 ml) skim milk	1 fat-free milk and yogurt

5,100- to 5,500-Calorie Meal Plan

Food group	Food group choices	Calorie level and number of choices
Fat-free milk and yogurt	8 oz (240 ml) fat-free or 1% milk 8 oz (240 ml) soy milk 8 oz (240 ml) low-fat kefir 6 oz (180 g) fat-free yogurt	5,100 kcal: choose 4 5,200 kcal: choose 4 5,300 kcal: choose 4 5,400 kcal: choose 4 5,500 kcal: choose 4
Nonstarchy vegetables	1 cup (56 g) dark green lettuce 15 raw baby carrots 1 large tomato 1/2 cup (62 g) cooked green beans 1/2 cup (78 g) cooked broccoli 1/2 cup (62 g) cooked cauliflower 1/2 cup (90 g) cooked zucchini 1 medium onion 1 bell pepper	5,100 kcal: choose 6 5,200 kcal: choose 6 5,300 kcal: choose 6 5,400 kcal: choose 6 5,500 kcal: choose 6
Fruits	1 small apple 1 small banana 1 cup (144 g) berries 1 small orange 2 tbsp (18 g) raisins 1/2 cup (120 ml) 100% fruit juice 17 grapes 1/2 cup (122 g) unsweetened applesauce 1/2 cup (128 g) cut fresh or canned fruit, unsweetened	5,100 kcal: choose 15 5,200 kcal: choose 15 5,300 kcal: choose 15 5,400 kcal: choose 15 5,500 kcal: choose 15
Grains and starches	1 slice bread 1/2 6-in. (15 cm) pita 1/2 English muffin 1/2 small (2 oz or 60 g) bagel 1/4 large (4 oz or 120 g) bagel 1/2 cup (121 g) cooked cereal 3/4 cup (21 g) unsweetened ready-to-eat cereal 1 4-in. (10 cm) thin pancake 1 4-in. (10 cm) square waffle 1/2 cup (93 g) cooked rice 1/2 cup (70 g) cooked pasta 1/3 cup (83 g) baked beans 1/2 cup (82 g) corn 1/4 large (3 oz or 90 g) potato 1 small dinner roll 3 graham cracker squares	5,100 kcal: choose 21 5,200 kcal: choose 22 5,300 kcal: choose 23 5,400 kcal: choose 23 5,500 kcal: choose 24
Foods with sugar	1 energy or granola bar (~1 oz or 30 g) 1 frozen 100% fruit juice bar 1 tbsp (21 g) honey, jam, or syrup or 1 tbsp (12 g) sugar 1 cup (8 oz or 240 ml) sports drink 1/2 cup (87 g) frozen yogurt	5,100 kcal: choose 9 5,200 kcal: choose 9 5,300 kcal: choose 9 5,400 kcal: choose 10 5,500 kcal: choose 10

Lean protein	1 oz (30 g) (very thin slice) *lean*
	   chicken
	   turkey
	   beef
	   pork
	   fish
	2 egg whites or 1/4 cup (61 g) egg substitute
		5,100 kcal: choose 10
		5,200 kcal: choose 10
		5,300 kcal: choose 10
		5,400 kcal: choose 11
		5,500 kcal: choose 11

Fats and oils	1 tsp (5 g) margarine 1 tbsp (15 g) reduced-fat margarine 1 tsp (5 g) oil 1 tsp (5 g) mayo 1 tbsp (14 g) reduced-fat mayo 1/2 tbsp (8 g) peanut or almond butter 1 tbsp (14 g) cream cheese 1 tbsp (16 g) salad dressing 2 tbsp (29 g) avocado 6 almonds 4 walnut halves 10 peanuts	5,100 kcal: choose 24 5,200 kcal: choose 25 5,300 kcal: choose 25 5,400 kcal: choose 26 5,500 kcal: choose 26

5,600- to 6,000-Calorie Meal Plan

Food group	Food group choices	Calorie level and number of choices
Fat-free milk and yogurt	8 oz (240 ml) fat-free or 1% milk 8 oz (240 ml) soy milk 8 oz (240 ml) low-fat kefir 6 oz (180 g) fat-free yogurt	5,600 kcal: choose 4 5,700 kcal: choose 4 5,800 kcal: choose 4 5,900 kcal: choose 4 6,000 kcal: choose 5
Nonstarchy vegetables	1 cup (56 g) dark green lettuce 15 raw baby carrots 1 large tomato 1/2 cup (62 g) cooked green beans 1/2 cup (78 g) cooked broccoli 1/2 cup (62 g) cooked cauliflower 1/2 cup (90 g) cooked zucchini 1 medium onion 1 bell pepper	5,600 kcal: choose 6 5,700 kcal: choose 6 5,800 kcal: choose 6 5,900 kcal: choose 6 6,000 kcal: choose 6
Fruits	1 small apple 1 small banana 1 cup (144 g) berries 1 small orange 2 tbsp (18 g) raisins 1/2 cup (120 ml) 100% fruit juice 17 grapes 1/2 cup (122 g) unsweetened applesauce 1/2 cup (128 g) cut fresh or canned fruit, unsweetened	5,600 kcal: choose 15 5,700 kcal: choose 16 5,800 kcal: choose 16 5,900 kcal: choose 17 6,000 kcal: choose 17
Grains and starches	1 slice bread 1/2 6-in. (15 cm) pita 1/2 English muffin 1/2 small (2 oz or 60 g) bagel 1/4 large (4 oz or 120 g) bagel 1/2 cup (121 g) cooked cereal 3/4 cup (21 g) unsweetened ready-to-eat cereal 1 4-in. (10 cm) thin pancake 1 4-in. (10 cm) square waffle 1/2 cup (93 g) cooked rice 1/2 cup (70 g) cooked pasta 1/3 cup (83 g) baked beans 1/2 cup (82 g) corn 1/4 large (3 oz or 90 g) potato 1 small dinner roll 3 graham cracker squares	5,600 kcal: choose 25 5,700 kcal: choose 25 5,800 kcal: choose 25 5,900 kcal: choose 26 6,000 kcal: choose 26
Foods with sugar	1 energy or granola bar (~1 oz or 30 g) 1 frozen 100% fruit juice bar 1 tbsp (21 g) honey, jam, or syrup or 1 tbsp (12 g) sugar 1 cup (8 oz or 240 ml) sports drink 1/2 cup (87 g) frozen yogurt	5,600 kcal: choose 10 5,700 kcal: choose 10 5,800 kcal: choose 11 5,900 kcal: choose 11 6,000 kcal: choose 11

Lean protein	1 oz (30 g) (very thin slice) *lean*
	    chicken
	    turkey
	    beef
	    pork
	    fish
	2 egg whites or 1/4 cup (61 g) egg substitute
		5,600 kcal: choose 11
		5,700 kcal: choose 11
		5,800 kcal: choose 12
		5,900 kcal: choose 12
		6,000 kcal: choose 12

Fats and oils	1 tsp (5 g) margarine 1 tbsp (15 g) reduced-fat margarine 1 tsp (5 g) oil 1 tsp (5 g) mayo 1 tbsp (14 g) reduced-fat mayo 1/2 tbsp (8 g) peanut or almond butter 1 tbsp (14 g) cream cheese 1 tbsp (16 g) salad dressing 2 tbsp (29 g) avocado 6 almonds 4 walnut halves 10 peanuts	5,600 kcal: choose 27 5,700 kcal: choose 27 5,800 kcal: choose 27 5,900 kcal: choose 27 6,000 kcal: choose 27

Sample 5,600-Calorie One-Day Menu

Meal or snack	Amount and food	Number of choices and food group
Breakfast	2 cups (484 g) cooked oatmeal	4 grains and starches
	4 tbsp (36 g) raisins	2 fruits
	1 tbsp (12 g) sugar	1 foods with sugar
	12 almonds	2 fats and oils
	1 English muffin	2 grains and starches
	4 tsp (20 g) margarine	4 fats and oils
	2 scrambled egg whites	1 lean protein
	8 oz (240 ml) orange juice	2 fruits
	8 oz (240 ml) skim milk	1 fat-free milk and yogurt
Lunch	4 slices whole-wheat bread	4 grains and starches
	4 slices (4 oz or 120 g) turkey breast	4 lean protein
	4 tsp (20 g) mayo	4 fats and oils
	4 tbsp (58 g) avocado	2 fats and oils
	Lettuce and tomato slices	1 nonstarchy vegetable
	2/3 cup (166 g) baked beans	2 grains and starches
	15 raw baby carrots	1 nonstarchy vegetable
	34 grapes	2 fruits
	1/2 cup (8 oz or 240 ml) 100% fruit juice	1 fruits
	8 oz (240 ml) skim milk	1 fat-free milk and yogurt
Preexercise snack	1 large banana	2 fruits
	1 1/2 cups (42 g) ready-to-eat cereal	2 grains and starches
	2 tbsp (18 g) raisins	1 fruits
	16 oz (480 ml) sports drink	2 foods with sugar
Postexercise snack	6 oz (180 g) fat-free yogurt	1 fat-free milk and yogurt
	1/2 cup (128 g) unsweetened canned fruit	1 fruits
	1 large orange	2 fruits
	9 squares graham crackers	3 grains and starches
	2 tbsp (48 g) peanut butter	4 fats and oils
	40 oz (1,200 ml) sports drink	5 foods with sugar
Dinner	6 oz (180 g) baked, skinless chicken breast	6 lean protein
	1 1/2 cup (246 g) corn	3 grains and starches
	1 cup baked beans (249 g)	3 grains and starches
	2 cups dark green lettuce (112 g)	2 nonstarchy vegetables
	1 bell pepper	1 nonstarchy vegetable
	1 large tomato	1 nonstarchy vegetable
	3 tbsp (48 g) salad dressing	3 fats and oils
	8 walnut halves	2 fats and oils
	2 whole-grain rolls	2 grains and starches
	6 tsp (25 g) margarine	6 fats and oils
	2 tbsp (42 g) honey	2 foods with sugar
	1 cup (244 g) unsweetened applesauce	2 fruits
	8 oz (240 ml) skim milk	1 fat-free milk and yogurt

6,100- to 6,500-Calorie Meal Plan

Food group	Food group choices	Calorie level and number of choices
Fat-free milk and yogurt	8 oz (240 ml) fat-free or 1% milk 8 oz (240 ml) soy milk 8 oz (240 ml) low-fat kefir 6 oz (180 g) fat-free yogurt	6,100 kcal: choose 5 6,200 kcal: choose 5 6,300 kcal: choose 5 6,400 kcal: choose 5 6,500 kcal: choose 5
Nonstarchy vegetables	1 cup (56 g) dark green lettuce 15 raw baby carrots 1 large tomato 1/2 cup (62 g) cooked green beans 1/2 cup (78 g) cooked broccoli 1/2 cup (62 g) cooked cauliflower 1/2 cup (90 g) cooked zucchini 1 medium onion 1 bell pepper	6,100 kcal: choose 6 6,200 kcal: choose 6 6,300 kcal: choose 6 6,400 kcal: choose 6 6,500 kcal: choose 6
Fruits	1 small apple 1 small banana 1 cup (144 g) berries 1 small orange 2 tbsp (18 g) raisins 1/2 cup (120 ml) 100% fruit juice 17 grapes 1/2 cup (122 g) unsweetened applesauce 1/2 cup (128 g) cut fresh or canned fruit, unsweetened	6,100 kcal: choose 18 6,200 kcal: choose 18 6,300 kcal: choose 18 6,400 kcal: choose 18 6,500 kcal: choose 18
Grains and starches	1 slice bread 1/2 6-in. (15 cm) pita 1/2 English muffin 1/2 small (2 oz or 60 g) bagel 1/4 large (4 oz or 120 g) bagel 1/2 cup (121 g) cooked cereal 3/4 cup (21 g) unsweetened ready-to-eat cereal 1 4-in. (10 cm) thin pancake 1 4-in. (10 cm) square waffle 1/2 cup (93 g) cooked rice 1/2 cup (70 g) cooked pasta 1/3 cup (83 g) baked beans 1/2 cup (82 g) corn 1/4 large (3 oz or 90 g) potato 1 small dinner roll 3 graham cracker squares	6,100 kcal: choose 26 6,200 kcal: choose 26 6,300 kcal: choose 26 6,400 kcal: choose 27 6,500 kcal: choose 28
Foods with sugar	1 energy or granola bar (~1 oz or 30 g) 1 frozen 100% fruit juice bar 1 tbsp (21 g) honey, jam, or syrup or 1 tbsp (12 g) sugar 1 cup (8 oz or 240 ml) sports drink 1/2 cup (87 g) frozen yogurt	6,100 kcal: choose 11 6,200 kcal: choose 12 6,300 kcal: choose 13 6,400 kcal: choose 13 6,500 kcal: choose 13

Lean protein	1 oz (30 g) (very thin slice) *lean*
	    chicken
	    turkey
	    beef
	    pork
	    fish
	2 egg whites or 1/4 cup (61 g) egg substitute
		6,100 kcal: choose 12
		6,200 kcal: choose 12
		6,300 kcal: choose 13
		6,400 kcal: choose 13
		6,500 kcal: choose 13

Fats and oils	1 tsp (5 g) margarine 1 tbsp (15 g) reduced-fat margarine 1 tsp (5 g) oil 1 tsp (5 g) mayo 1 tbsp (14 g) reduced-fat mayo 1/2 tbsp (8 g) peanut or almond butter 1 tbsp (14 g) cream cheese 1 tbsp (16 g) salad dressing 2 tbsp (29 g) avocado 6 almonds 4 walnut halves 10 peanuts	6,100 kcal: choose 28 6,200 kcal: choose 28 6,300 kcal: choose 28 6,400 kcal: choose 29 6,500 kcal: choose 29

6,600- to 7,000-Calorie Meal Plan

Food group	Food group choices	Calorie level and number of choices
Fat-free milk and yogurt	8 oz (240 ml) fat-free or 1% milk 8 oz (240 ml) soy milk 8 oz (240 ml) low-fat kefir 6 oz (180 g) fat-free yogurt	6,600 kcal: choose 5 6,700 kcal: choose 5 6,800 kcal: choose 5 6,900 kcal: choose 6 7,000 kcal: choose 6
Nonstarchy vegetables	1 cup (56 g) dark green lettuce 15 raw baby carrots 1 large tomato 1/2 cup (62 g) cooked green beans 1/2 cup (78 g) cooked broccoli 1/2 cup (62 g) cooked cauliflower 1/2 cup (90 g) cooked zucchini 1 medium onion 1 bell pepper	6,600 kcal: choose 6 6,700 kcal: choose 6 6,800 kcal: choose 6 6,900 kcal: choose 6 7,000 kcal: choose 6
Fruits	1 small apple 1 small banana 1 cup (144 g) berries 1 small orange 2 tbsp (18 g) raisins 1/2 cup (120 ml) 100% fruit juice 17 grapes 1/2 cup (122 g) unsweetened applesauce 1/2 cup (128 g) cut fresh or canned fruit, unsweetened	6,600 kcal: choose 18 6,700 kcal: choose 18 6,800 kcal: choose 18 6,900 kcal: choose 18 7,000 kcal: choose 18
Grains and starches	1 slice bread 1/2 6-in. (15 cm) pita 1/2 English muffin 1/2 small (2 oz or 60 g) bagel 1/4 large (4 oz or 120 g) bagel 1/2 cup (121 g) cooked cereal 3/4 cup (21 g) unsweetened ready-to-eat cereal 1 4-in. (10 cm) thin pancake 1 4-in. (10 cm) square waffle 1/2 cup (93 g) cooked rice 1/2 cup (70 g) cooked pasta 1/3 cup (83 g) baked beans 1/2 cup (82 g) corn 1/4 large (3 oz or 90 g) potato 1 small dinner roll 3 graham cracker squares	6,600 kcal: choose 29 6,700 kcal: choose 29 6,800 kcal: choose 29 6,900 kcal: choose 29 7,000 kcal: choose 29
Foods with sugar	1 energy or granola bar (~1 oz or 30 g) 1 frozen 100% fruit juice bar 1 tbsp (21 g) honey, jam, or syrup or 1 tbsp (12 g) sugar 1 cup (8 oz or 240 ml) sports drink 1/2 cup (87 g) frozen yogurt	6,600 kcal: choose 13 6,700 kcal: choose 14 6,800 kcal: choose 15 6,900 kcal: choose 15 7,000 kcal: choose 15

Lean protein	1 oz (30 g) (very thin slice) *lean*
	   chicken
	   turkey
	   beef
	   pork
	   fish
	2 egg whites or 1/4 cup (61 g) egg substitute
		6,600 kcal: choose 13
		6,700 kcal: choose 13
		6,800 kcal: choose 14
		6,900 kcal: choose 14
		7,000 kcal: choose 16

Fats and oils	1 tsp (5 g) margarine 1 tbsp (15 g) reduced-fat margarine 1 tsp (5 g) oil 1 tsp (5 g) mayo 1 tbsp (14 g) reduced-fat mayo 1/2 tbsp (8 g) peanut or almond butter 1 tbsp (14 g) cream cheese 1 tbsp (16 g) salad dressing 2 tbsp (29 g) avocado 6 almonds 4 walnut halves 10 peanuts	6,600 kcal: choose 30 6,700 kcal: choose 31 6,800 kcal: choose 31 6,900 kcal: choose 31 7,000 kcal: choose 31

Sample 6,600-Calorie One-Day Menu

Meal or snack	Amount and food	Number of choices and food group
Breakfast	2 cups (484 g) cooked oatmeal	4 grains and starches
	4 tbsp (36 g) raisins	2 fruits
	1 tbsp (12 g) brown sugar	1 foods with sugar
	12 almonds	2 fats and oils
	2 tsp (10 g) margarine	2 fats and oils
	1 (4 oz or 120 g) bagel	4 grains and starches
	2 tbsp (28 g) cream cheese	2 fats and oils
	1 tbsp (21 g) jam	1 foods with sugar
	4 scrambled egg whites	2 lean protein
	8 oz (240 ml) orange juice	2 fruits
	16 oz (480 ml) skim milk	2 fat-free milk and yogurt
Lunch	4 slices whole-wheat bread	4 grains and starches
	4 slices (4 oz or 120 g) turkey breast	4 lean protein
	5 tsp (25 g) mayo	5 fats and oils
	6 tbsp (87 g) avocado	3 fats and oils
	Lettuce and tomato slices	1 nonstarchy vegetable
	2/3 cup (166 g) baked beans	2 grains and starches
	15 raw baby carrots	1 nonstarchy vegetable
	34 grapes	2 fruits
	1 cup (8 oz or 240 ml) 100% fruit juice	2 fruits
	6 oz (180 g) fat-free yogurt	1 fat-free milk and yogurt
Preexercise snack	1 large banana	2 fruits
	2 1/4 cups (63 g) ready-to-eat cereal	3 grains and starches
	2 tbsp (18 g) raisins	1 fruits
	16 oz (480 ml) sports drink	2 foods with sugar
Postexercise snack	8 oz (1 cup or 240 ml) low-fat kefir	1 fat-free milk and yogurt
	1/2 cup (128 g) unsweetened canned fruit	1 fruits
	1 large orange	2 fruits
	1 large (4 oz or 120 g) bagel	4 grains and starches
	2 tbsp (48 g) peanut butter	4 fats and oils
	2 oz (60 g) energy bar	2 foods with sugar
	40 oz (1,200 ml) sports drink	5 foods with sugar
Dinner	7 oz (200 g) baked, skinless chicken breast	7 lean protein
	1 1/2 cup (246 g) corn	3 grains and starches
	1 cup (249 g) baked beans	3 grains and starches
	2 cups (112 g) dark green lettuce	2 nonstarchy vegetables
	1 bell pepper	1 nonstarchy vegetable
	1 large tomato	1 nonstarchy vegetable
	3 tbsp (48 g) salad dressing	3 fats and oils
	12 walnut halves	3 fats and oils
	2 whole-grain rolls	2 grains and starches
	6 tsp (25 g) margarine	6 fats and oils
	2 tbsp (42 g) honey	2 foods with sugar
	1 cup (244 g) unsweetened applesauce	2 fruits
	2 cups (288 g) berries	2 fruits
	8 oz (1 cup or 240 ml) skim milk	1 fat-free milk and yogurt

Losing Fat

This chapter is for athletes who want to lose body fat and decrease total weight. (If you want to gain muscle, refer to chapter 10. If your goal is to lose fat *and* build muscle, see chapter 12.) Many recreational athletes have the goal of losing weight, particularly those who participate in sports like marathons and triathlons that require them to move their bodies over a long distance. Well-trained athletes may want to decrease body fat if excess weight is hampering speed, negatively affecting endurance, or interfering with good health.

To meet your goal of losing body fat, you must do three things:

- Consume the correct number of calories
- Consume protein, carbohydrate, and fat in the appropriate amounts and proportions
- Engage in additional activity daily without overtraining

The first step to achieve your goal of losing fat is to determine the number of calories that you need on a daily basis. If your current body weight is stable, you can use the figures that you obtained in calculating your average daily caloric intake (chapter 3). Thus, your current intake is your baseline.

If you are currently gaining weight, then you should calculate your estimated caloric need as explained in chapter 5. This estimate will become your baseline so it must be as accurate as possible. You must evaluate your progress regularly to assess whether you are within an appropriate calorie range to lose body fat and be prepared to adjust as needed.

After you have found your baseline calorie intake, decide on a calorie decrease as shown in table 11.1. As a starting point, males generally decrease their caloric intake by 300 to 500 kilocalories daily and females by 200 to 300 kilocalories daily. Remember that although you must moderately reduce your calories daily, the reduction cannot be too severe because you still need enough calories to support your training and prevent a decrease in metabolic rate. Consuming too few calories can slow your rate of fat loss rather than accelerate it!

TABLE 11.1

Calories Needed to Lose Fat

Goal	Gender	Total calories
To lose body fat	Male	Baseline kcal minus 300 to 500 kcal
	Female	Baseline kcal minus 200 to 300 kcal

Select Your Jumpstart Meal Plan

After you have determined how many calories you need to lose body fat, you are ready to choose a jumpstart meal plan for that calorie level. The simple plans in this chapter are intended to jump-start your effort to lose body fat. Adherence to these plans will establish a pattern of eating that will help you achieve your body-composition and performance goals.

Because the plans offer a limited number of food choices, they are easy to follow. The drawback of this simplicity is a lack of variety, so you should not use these plans for more than a week or two. A monotonous diet is difficult to follow for long, and the lack of variety limits your nutrient intake. After the initial period, you should create a customized, personal plan to expand the range of foods that you consume. Following the precision meal planning system in chapter 13 makes customization easy. Creating a diet with your favorite foods and with a greater variety of foods means that you will be able to follow your customized plan over the months required to meet your goals.

Each meal plan contains the proper amount and proportions of carbohydrate, protein, and fat to help maintain muscle mass while supporting maximum fat loss. The plans have been designed to contain approximately 5 grams of carbohydrate per kilogram of body weight so that you will have enough carbohydrate to replenish the muscle glycogen used during exercise. To help protect against loss of lean body mass, the meal plans contain about 1.5 grams of protein per kilogram of body weight. The remainder of the calories comes from fat in sufficient quantity to help satisfy appetite.

Each meal plan consists of seven food groups and indicates the total number of choices that you should make from each group. Within each food group you may choose any foods that you like, but to maintain the right calorie level and macronutrient balance, you need to consume the quantities specified. If you yield to the temptation of eating less than recommended, you will not be consuming the nutrients that you need for training and recovery, and you may unwittingly reduce your metabolic rate.

Select the plan that is right for you by following these simple steps:

1. Select the correct calorie range for your needs based on table 11.1. The meal plans are provided in 500 kilocalorie increments. For example, if you need 2,200 kilocalories daily, refer to the 1,900 to 2,300 kilocalories meal plan.

2. Choose the right number of foods from each food group for your calorie level. For example, a 2,200-kilocalorie diet consists of three choices from the fat-free milk and yogurt group, four choices from the nonstarchy vegetables group, and so on. When you need to choose more than one food from a group, you can select any combination to reach the total number of choices. You may choose any food listed more than once. For example, three fat-free milk and yogurt choices could be three 8-ounce (240-milliliter) glasses of fat-free milk or one 8-ounce (240-milliliter) glass of soy milk, one 8-ounce (240-milliliter) glass of low-fat kefir, and 6 ounces (180 grams) of fat-free yogurt. In choosing among the options in each food group, remember not to exceed the total number of choices for the day.

3. Create three meals and two snacks from the foods chosen. Eat the snacks before and after you exercise.

Four sample menus illustrate how to translate the number of choices in the meal plan into meals and snacks. (See chapter 13 for additional information about how to create meals and snacks.) The meals and snacks that you create may look different from these sample menus because you have several choices in each food group. When you divide the total choices in your meal plan into meals and snacks, remember that you should have at least three meals and two snacks each day. When trying to lose body fat, you should eat small amounts throughout the day. Skipping meals often leads to excessive hunger and overeating. For proper recovery, consume some carbohydrate and protein in the first hour after exercise (see chapter 6).

1,900- to 2,300-Calorie Meal Plan

Food group	Food group choices	Calorie level and number of choices
Fat-free milk and yogurt	8 oz (240 ml) fat-free or 1% milk 8 oz (240 ml) soy milk 8 oz (240 ml) low-fat kefir 6 oz (180 g) fat-free yogurt	1,900 kcal: choose 2 2,000 kcal: choose 2 2,100 kcal: choose 2 2,200 kcal: choose 3 2,300 kcal: choose 3
Nonstarchy vegetables	1 cup (56 g) dark green lettuce 15 raw baby carrots 1 large tomato 1/2 cup (62 g) cooked green beans 1/2 cup (78 g) cooked broccoli 1/2 cup (62 g) cooked cauliflower 1/2 cup (90 g) cooked zucchini 1 medium onion 1 bell pepper	1,900 kcal: choose 4 2,000 kcal: choose 4 2,100 kcal: choose 4 2,200 kcal: choose 4 2,300 kcal: choose 4
Fruits	1 small apple 1 small banana 1 cup (144 g) berries 1 small orange 2 tbsp (18 g) raisins 1/2 cup (120 ml) 100% fruit juice 17 grapes 1/2 cup (122 g) unsweetened applesauce 1/2 cup (128 g) cut fresh or canned fruit, unsweetened	1,900 kcal: choose 8 2,000 kcal: choose 8 2,100 kcal: choose 9 2,200 kcal: choose 9 2,300 kcal: choose 9
Grains and starches	1 slice bread 1/2 6-in. (15 cm) pita 1/2 English muffin 1/2 small (2 oz or 60 g) bagel 1/4 large (4 oz or 120 g) bagel 1/2 cup (121 g) cooked cereal 3/4 cup (21 g) unsweetened ready-to-eat cereal 1 4-in. (10 cm) thin pancake 1 4-in. (10 cm) square waffle 1/2 cup (93 g) cooked rice 1/2 cup (70 g) cooked pasta 1/3 cup (83 g) baked beans 1/2 cup (82 g) corn 1/4 large (3 oz or 90 g) potato 1 small dinner roll 3 graham cracker squares	1,900 kcal: choose 6 2,000 kcal: choose 7 2,100 kcal: choose 7 2,200 kcal: choose 7 2,300 kcal: choose 8
Foods with sugar	None*	1,900 kcal: choose 0 2,000 kcal: choose 0 2,100 kcal: choose 0 2,200 kcal: choose 0 2,300 kcal: choose 0

Lean protein	1 oz (30 g) (very thin slice) *lean*
	    chicken
	    turkey
	    beef
	    pork
	    fish
	2 egg whites or 1/4 cup (61 g) egg substitute
		1,900 kcal: choose 5
		2,000 kcal: choose 5
		2,100 kcal: choose 5
		2,200 kcal: choose 5
		2,300 kcal: choose 5

Fats and oils	1 tsp (5 g) margarine 1 tbsp (15 g) reduced-fat margarine 1 tsp (5 g) oil 1 tsp (5 g) mayo 1 tbsp (14 g) reduced-fat mayo 1/2 tbsp (8 g) peanut or almond butter 1 tbsp (14 g) cream cheese 1 tbsp (16 g) salad dressing 2 tbsp (29 g) avocado 6 almonds 4 walnut halves 10 peanuts	1,900 kcal: choose 9 2,000 kcal: choose 10 2,100 kcal: choose 11 2,200 kcal: choose 11 2,300 kcal: choose 12

*The calorie intake levels for this meal plan do not allow consumption of foods with sugar.

Sample 1,900-Calorie One-Day Menu

Meal or snack	Amount and food	Number of choices and food group
Breakfast	3/4 cup (21 g) unsweetened ready-to-eat cereal	1 grains and starches
	1 small banana	1 fruits
	1/2 English muffin	1 grains and starches
	1/2 tbsp (8 g) almond butter	1 fats and oils
	1/2 cup (120 ml) orange juice	1 fruits
	8 oz (1 cup, or 240 ml) skim milk	1 fat-free milk and yogurt
Lunch	1 whole-wheat pita bread	2 grains and starches
	2 oz (60 g) chicken breast	2 lean protein
	Spinach leaves, sliced tomato, and sliced cucumber	1 nonstarchy vegetable
	1 tbsp (14 g) reduced-fat mayo (add mustard if desired)	1 fats and oils
	4 walnut halves	1 fats and oils
	1 small apple	1 fruits
	Calorie-free beverage	
Preexercise snack	1 small banana	1 fruits
	1/2 cup (120 ml) 100% fruit juice	1 fruits
Postexercise snack	8 oz (1 cup, or 240 ml) low-fat kefir	1 fat-free milk and yogurt
	1 medium-large apple	2 fruits
	1 1/2 tbsp (24 g) peanut butter	3 fats and oils
Dinner	3 oz (90 g) grilled salmon	3 lean protein
	1/2 cup (78 g) cooked broccoli	1 nonstarchy vegetable
	1/2 large (6 oz or 180 g) potato	2 grains and starches
	1 cup (56 g) dark green lettuce	1 nonstarchy vegetable
	1 cup (150 g) chopped raw pepper, tomato, carrot	1 nonstarchy vegetable
	4 walnut halves	1 fats and oils
	2 tbsp (32 g) salad dressing	2 fats and oils
	1/2 cup (128 g) cut fresh fruit	1 fruits
	Calorie-free beverage	

2,400- to 2,800-Calorie Meal Plans

Food group	Food group choices	Calorie level and number of choices
Fat-free milk and yogurt	8 oz (240 ml) fat-free or 1% milk 8 oz (240 ml) soy milk 8 oz (240 ml) low-fat kefir 6 oz (180 g) fat-free yogurt	2,400 kcal: choose 3 2,500 kcal: choose 3 2,600 kcal: choose 3 2,700 kcal: choose 3 2,800 kcal: choose 3
Nonstarchy vegetables	1 cup (56 g) dark green lettuce 15 raw baby carrots 1 large tomato 1/2 cup (62 g) cooked green beans 1/2 cup (78 g) cooked broccoli 1/2 cup (62 g) cooked cauliflower 1/2 cup (90 g) cooked zucchini 1 medium onion 1 bell pepper	2,400 kcal: choose 4 2,500 kcal: choose 4 2,600 kcal: choose 5 2,700 kcal: choose 5 2,800 kcal: choose 5
Fruits	1 small apple 1 small banana 1 cup (144 g) berries 1 small orange 2 tbsp (18 g) raisins 1/2 cup (120 ml) 100% fruit juice 17 grapes 1/2 cup (122 g) unsweetened applesauce 1/2 cup (128 g) cut fresh or canned fruit, unsweetened	2,400 kcal: choose 10 2,500 kcal: choose 10 2,600 kcal: choose 10 2,700 kcal: choose 10 2,800 kcal: choose 10
Grains and starches	1 slice bread 1/2 6-in. (15 cm) pita 1/2 English muffin 1/2 small (2 oz or 60 g) bagel 1/4 large (4 oz or 120 g) bagel 1/2 cup (121 g) cooked cereal 3/4 cup (21 g) unsweetened ready-to-eat cereal 1 4-in. (10 cm) thin pancake 1 4-in. (10 cm) square waffle 1/2 cup (93 g) cooked rice 1/2 cup (70 g) cooked pasta 1/3 cup (83 g) baked beans 1/2 cup (82 g) corn 1/4 large (3 oz or 90 g) potato 1 small dinner roll 3 graham cracker squares	2,400 kcal: choose 8 2,500 kcal: choose 9 2,600 kcal: choose 9 2,700 kcal: choose 9 2,800 kcal: choose 10
Foods with sugar	1 energy or granola bar (~1 oz or 30 g) 1 frozen 100% fruit juice bar 1 tbsp (21 g) honey, jam, or syrup or 1 tbsp (12 g) sugar 1 cup (8 oz or 240 ml) sports drink 1/2 cup (87 g) frozen yogurt	2,400 kcal: choose 0 2,500 kcal: choose 0 2,600 kcal: choose 0 2,700 kcal: choose 1 2,800 kcal: choose 1

Lean protein	1 oz (30 g) (very thin slice) *lean*
	    chicken
	    turkey
	    beef
	    pork
	    fish
	2 egg whites or 1/4 cup (61 g) egg substitute
		2,400 kcal: choose 6
		2,500 kcal: choose 6
		2,600 kcal: choose 6
		2,700 kcal: choose 7
		2,800 kcal: choose 7

Fats and oils	1 tsp (5 g) margarine 1 tbsp (15 g) reduced-fat margarine 1 tsp (5 g) oil 1 tsp (5 g) mayo 1 tbsp (14 g) reduced-fat mayo 1/2 tbsp (8 g) peanut or almond butter 1 tbsp (14 g) cream cheese 1 tbsp (16 g) salad dressing 2 tbsp (29 g) avocado 6 almonds 4 walnut halves 10 peanuts	2,400 kcal: choose 12 2,500 kcal: choose 13 2,600 kcal: choose 14 2,700 kcal: choose 14 2,800 kcal: choose 14

2,900- to 3,300-Calorie Meal Plans

Food group	Food group choices	Calorie level and number of choices
Fat-free milk and yogurt	8 oz (240 ml) fat-free or 1% milk 8 oz (240 ml) soy milk 8 oz (240 ml) low-fat kefir 6 oz (180 g) fat-free yogurt	2,900 kcal: choose 3 3,000 kcal: choose 3 3,100 kcal: choose 3 3,200 kcal: choose 3 3,300 kcal: choose 3
Nonstarchy vegetables	1 cup (56 g) dark green lettuce 15 raw baby carrots 1 large tomato 1/2 cup (62 g) cooked green beans 1/2 cup (78 g) cooked broccoli 1/2 cup (62 g) cooked cauliflower 1/2 cup (90 g) cooked zucchini 1 medium onion 1 bell pepper	2,900 kcal: choose 5 3,000 kcal: choose 5 3,100 kcal: choose 5 3,200 kcal: choose 5 3,300 kcal: choose 5
Fruits	1 small apple 1 small banana 1 cup (144 g) berries 1 small orange 2 tbsp (18 g) raisins 1/2 cup (120 ml) 100% fruit juice 17 grapes 1/2 cup (122 g) unsweetened applesauce 1/2 cup (128 g) cut fresh or canned fruit, unsweetened	2,900 kcal: choose 11 3,000 kcal: choose 11 3,100 kcal: choose 11 3,200 kcal: choose 11 3,300 kcal: choose 11
Grains and starches	1 slice bread 1/2 6-in. (15 cm) pita 1/2 English muffin 1/2 small (2 oz or 30 g) bagel 1/4 large (4 oz or 120 g) bagel 1/2 cup (121 g) cooked cereal 3/4 cup (21 g) unsweetened ready-to-eat cereal 1 4-in. (10 cm) thin pancake 1 4-in. (10 cm) square waffle 1/2 cup (93 g) cooked rice 1/2 cup (70 g) cooked pasta 1/3 cup (83 g) baked beans 1/2 cup (82 g) corn 1/4 large (3 oz or 90 g) potato 1 small dinner roll 3 graham cracker squares	2,900 kcal: choose 10 3,000 kcal: choose 10 3,100 kcal: choose 11 3,200 kcal: choose 11 3,300 kcal: choose 12
Foods with sugar	1 energy or granola bar (~1 oz or 30 g) 1 frozen 100% fruit juice bar 1 tbsp (21 g) honey, jam, or syrup or 1 tbsp (12 g) sugar 1 cup (8 oz or 240 ml) sports drink 1/2 cup (87 g) frozen yogurt	2,900 kcal: choose 1 3,000 kcal: choose 2 3,100 kcal: choose 2 3,200 kcal: choose 3 3,300 kcal: choose 3

Lean protein	1 oz (30 g) (very thin slice) *lean*
	   chicken
	   turkey
	   beef
	   pork
	   fish
	2 egg whites or 1/4 cup (61 g) egg substitute
		2,900 kcal: choose 7
		3,000 kcal: choose 8
		3,100 kcal: choose 8
		3,200 kcal: choose 9
		3,300 kcal: choose 9

Fats and oils	1 tsp (5 g) margarine 1 tbsp (15 g) reduced-fat margarine 1 tsp (5 g) oil 1 tsp (5 g) mayo 1 tbsp (14 g) reduced-fat mayo 1/2 tbsp (8 g) peanut or almond butter 1 tbsp (14 g) cream cheese 1 tbsp (16 g) salad dressing 2 tbsp (29 g) avocado 6 almonds 4 walnut halves 10 peanuts	2,900 kcal: choose 15 3,000 kcal: choose 15 3,100 kcal: choose 15 3,200 kcal: choose 16 3,300 kcal: choose 16

Sample 2,900-Calorie One-Day Menu

Meal or snack	Amount and food	Number of choices and food group
Breakfast	3/4 cup (21 g) unsweetened ready-to-eat cereal	1 grains and starches
	1 small banana	1 fruits
	1 English muffin	2 grains and starches
	1 tbsp (16 g) almond butter	2 fats and oils
	1/2 cup (120 ml) orange juice	1 fruits
	8 oz (1 cup or 240 ml) skim milk	1 fat-free milk and yogurt
Lunch	1 whole-wheat pita bread	2 grains and starches
	3 oz (90 g) chicken breast	3 lean protein
	Spinach leaves, sliced tomato and sliced cucumber	1 nonstarchy vegetable
	1 tbsp (14 g) reduced-fat mayo (add mustard if desired)	1 fats and oils
	8 walnut halves	2 fats and oils
	1 small apple	1 fruits
	1 large orange	2 fruits
Preexercise snack	1 small banana	1 fruits
	4 oz (1/2 cup or 120 ml) 100% fruit juice	1 fruits
	6 squares graham crackers	2 grains and starches
Postexercise snack	8 oz (1 cup or 240 ml) low-fat kefir	1 fat-free milk and yogurt
	1 medium-large apple	2 fruits
	2 tbsp (40 g) peanut butter	4 fats and oils
	3 squares graham crackers	1 grains and starches
	8 oz (1 cup, or 240 ml) sports drink	1 foods with sugar
Dinner	4 oz (120 g) grilled salmon	4 lean protein
	1/2 cup (78 g) cooked broccoli	1 nonstarchy vegetable
	1/2 large (6 oz or 90 g) potato	2 grains and starches
	2 cup (112 g) dark green lettuce	2 nonstarchy vegetable
	1 cup (150 g) chopped raw pepper, tomato, carrot	1 nonstarchy vegetable
	8 walnut halves	2 fats and oils
	2 tbsp (32 g) salad dressing	2 fats and oils
	2 tsp (10 g) margarine	2 fats and oils
	1 cup (256 g) cut fresh fruit	2 fruits
	8 oz (1 cup or 240 ml) skim milk	1 fat-free milk and yogurt

3,400- to 3,800-Calorie Meal Plan

Food group	Food group choices	Calorie level and number of choices
Fat-free milk and yogurt	8 oz (240 ml) fat-free or 1% milk 8 oz (240 ml) soy milk 8 oz (240 ml) low-fat kefir 6 oz (180 g) fat-free yogurt	3,400 kcal: choose 3 3,500 kcal: choose 3 3,600 kcal: choose 3 3,700 kcal: choose 3 3,800 kcal: choose 3
Nonstarchy vegetables	1 cup (56 g) dark green lettuce 15 raw baby carrots 1 large tomato 1/2 cup (62 g) cooked green beans 1/2 cup (78 g) cooked broccoli 1/2 cup (62 g) cooked cauliflower 1/2 cup (90 g) cooked zucchini 1 medium onion 1 bell pepper	3,400 kcal: choose 6 3,500 kcal: choose 6 3,600 kcal: choose 6 3,700 kcal: choose 6 3,800 kcal: choose 8
Fruits	1 small apple 1 small banana 1 cup (144 g) berries 1 small orange 2 tbsp (18 g) raisins 1/2 cup (120 ml) 100% fruit juice 17 grapes 1/2 cup (122 g) unsweetened applesauce 1/2 cup (128 g) cut fresh or canned fruit, unsweetened	3,400 kcal: choose 11 3,500 kcal: choose 11 3,600 kcal: choose 12 3,700 kcal: choose 12 3,800 kcal: choose 12
Grains and starches	1 slice bread 1/2 6-in. (15 cm) pita 1/2 English muffin 1/2 small (2 oz or 60 g) bagel 1/4 large (4 oz or 120 g) bagel 1/2 cup (121 g) cooked cereal 3/4 cup (21 g) unsweetened ready-to-eat cereal 1 4-in. (10 cm) thin pancake 1 4-in. (10 cm) square waffle 1/2 cup (93 g) cooked rice 1/2 cup (70 g) cooked pasta 1/3 cup (83 g) baked beans 1/2 cup (82 g) corn 1/4 large (3 oz or 90 g) potato 1 small dinner roll 3 graham cracker squares	3,400 kcal: choose 12 3,500 kcal: choose 13 3,600 kcal: choose 13 3,700 kcal: choose 14 3,800 kcal: choose 14
Foods with sugar	1 energy or granola bar (~1 oz or 30 g) 1 frozen 100% fruit juice bar 1 tbsp (21 g) honey, jam, or syrup or 1 tbsp (12 g) sugar 1 cup (8 oz or 240 ml) sports drink 1/2 cup (87 g) frozen yogurt	3,400 kcal: choose 3 3,500 kcal: choose 3 3,600 kcal: choose 3 3,700 kcal: choose 3 3,800 kcal: choose 3

Lean protein	1 oz (30 g) (very thin slice) *lean*
	   chicken
	   turkey
	   beef
	   pork
	   fish
	2 egg whites or 1/4 cup (61 g) egg substitute
		3,400 kcal: choose 9
		3,500 kcal: choose 9
		3,600 kcal: choose 10
		3,700 kcal: choose 10
		3,800 kcal: choose 10

Fats and oils	1 tsp (5 g) margarine 1 tbsp (15 g) reduced-fat margarine 1 tsp (5 g) oil 1 tsp (5 g) mayo 1 tbsp (14 g) reduced-fat mayo 1/2 tbsp (8 g) peanut or almond butter 1 tbsp (14 g) cream cheese 1 tbsp (16 g) salad dressing 2 tbsp (29 g) avocado 6 almonds 4 walnut halves 10 peanuts	3,400 kcal: choose 17 3,500 kcal: choose 18 3,600 kcal: choose 18 3,700 kcal: choose 18 3,800 kcal: choose 19

3,900- to 4,300-Calorie Meal Plans

Food group	Food group choices	Calorie level and number of choices
Fat-free milk and yogurt	8 oz (240 ml) fat-free or 1% milk 8 oz (240 ml) soy milk 8 oz (240 ml) low-fat kefir 6 oz (180 g) fat-free yogurt	3,900 kcal: choose 3 4,000 kcal: choose 3 4,100 kcal: choose 3 4,200 kcal: choose 3 4,300 kcal: choose 3
Nonstarchy vegetables	1 cup (56 g) dark green lettuce 15 raw baby carrots 1 large tomato 1/2 cup (62 g) cooked green beans 1/2 cup (78 g) cooked broccoli 1/2 cup (62 g) cooked cauliflower 1/2 cup (90 g) cooked zucchini 1 medium onion 1 bell pepper	3,900 kcal: choose 7 4,000 kcal: choose 7 4,100 kcal: choose 8 4,200 kcal: choose 8 4,300 kcal: choose 8
Fruits	1 small apple 1 small banana 1 cup (144 g) berries 1 small orange 2 tbsp (18 g) raisins 1/2 cup (120 ml) 100% fruit juice 17 grapes 1/2 cup (122 g) unsweetened applesauce 1/2 cup (128 g) cut fresh or canned fruit, unsweetened	3,900 kcal: choose 12 4,000 kcal: choose 12 4,100 kcal: choose 12 4,200 kcal: choose 12 4,300 kcal: choose 12
Grains and starches	1 slice bread 1/2 6-in. (15 cm) pita 1/2 English muffin 1/2 small (2 oz or 60 g) bagel 1/4 large (4 oz or 120 g) bagel 1/2 cup (121 g) cooked cereal 3/4 cup (21 g) unsweetened ready-to-eat cereal 1 4-in. (10 cm) thin pancake 1 4-in. (10 cm) square waffle 1/2 cup (93 g) cooked rice 1/2 cup (70 g) cooked pasta 1/3 cup (83 g) baked beans 1/2 cup (82 g) corn 1/4 large (3 oz or 90 g) potato 1 small dinner roll 3 graham cracker squares	3,900 kcal: choose 15 4,000 kcal: choose 15 4,100 kcal: choose 16 4,200 kcal: choose 17 4,300 kcal: choose 17
Foods with sugar	1 energy or granola bar (~1 oz or 30 g) 1 frozen 100% fruit juice bar 1 tbsp (21 g) honey, jam, or syrup or 1 tbsp (12 g) sugar 1 cup (8 oz or 240 ml) sports drink 1/2 cup (87 g) frozen yogurt	3,900 kcal: choose 3 4,000 kcal: choose 4 4,100 kcal: choose 4 4,200 kcal: choose 4 4,300 kcal: choose 4

Lean protein	1 oz (30 g) (very thin slice) *lean*
	    chicken
	    turkey
	    beef
	    pork
	    fish
	2 egg whites or 1/4 cup (61 g) egg substitute
		3,900 kcal: choose 11
		4,000 kcal: choose 11
		4,100 kcal: choose 11
		4,200 kcal: choose 11
		4,300 kcal: choose 12

Fats and oils	1 tsp (5 g) margarine 1 tbsp (15 g) reduced-fat margarine 1 tsp (5 g) oil 1 tsp (5 g) mayo 1 tbsp (14 g) reduced-fat mayo 1/2 tbsp (8 g) peanut or almond butter 1 tbsp (14 g) cream cheese 1 tbsp (16 g) salad dressing 2 tbsp (29 g) avocado 6 almonds 4 walnut halves 10 peanuts	3,900 kcal: choose 19 4,000 kcal: choose 20 4,100 kcal: choose 20 4,200 kcal: choose 21 4,300 kcal: choose 21

Sample 3,900-Calorie One-Day Menu

Meal or snack	Amount and food	Number of choices and food group
Breakfast	1 1/2 cups (42 g) unsweetened ready-to-eat cereal	2 grains and starches
	1 small banana	1 fruits
	1 whole-grain English muffin	2 grains and starches
	2 tsp (10 g) margarine	2 fats and oils
	1 tsp honey	1 foods with sugar
	2 scrambled egg whites or 1/4 cup egg substitute	1 lean protein
	8 oz (1 cup or 240 ml) orange juice	2 fruits
	8 oz (1 cup or 240 ml) skim milk	1 fat-free milk and yogurt
Lunch	1 whole-wheat pita bread	2 grains and starches
	4 oz (120 g) chicken breast	4 lean protein
	Spinach leaves, sliced tomato, and sliced cucumber	1 nonstarchy vegetables
	8 raw baby carrots and 1/2 bell pepper	1 nonstarchy vegetables
	2 tbsp (28 g) reduced-fat mayo	2 fats and oils
	8 walnut halves	2 fats and oils
	1 small apple	1 fruits
	1 large orange	2 fruits
Preexercise snack	1 large banana	2 fruits
	6 squares graham crackers	2 grains and starches
	8 oz (1 cup or 240 ml) sports drink	1 foods with sugar
Postexercise snack	8 oz (1 cup or 240 ml) low-fat kefir	1 fat-free milk and yogurt
	4 tbsp (36 g) raisins	2 fruits
	50 peanuts	5 fats and oils
	2 1/4 cups (63 g) ready-to-eat cereal	3 grains and starches
	8 oz (1 cup or 240 ml) sports drink	1 foods with sugar
Dinner	6 oz (180 g) grilled salmon	6 lean protein
	1 cup (156 g) cooked broccoli	2 nonstarchy vegetables
	1 large (12 oz or 360 g) potato	4 grains and starches
	2 cups (112 g) dark green lettuce	2 nonstarchy vegetables
	1 cup (150 g) chopped raw pepper, tomato, carrot	1 nonstarchy vegetables
	12 walnut halves	3 fats and oils
	2 tbsp (32 g) salad dressing	2 fats and oils
	3 tsp (15 g) margarine	3 fats and oils
	1 cup (256 g) cut fresh fruit	2 fruits
	8 oz (1 cup or 240 ml) skim milk	1 fat-free milk and yogurt

4,400- to 4,900-Calorie Meal Plan

Food group	Food group choices	Calorie level and number of choices
Fat-free milk and yogurt	8 oz (240 ml) fat-free or 1% milk 8 oz (240 ml) soy milk 8 oz (240 ml) low-fat kefir 6 oz (180 g) fat-free yogurt	4,400 kcal: choose 3 4,500 kcal: choose 4 4,600 kcal: choose 4 4,700 kcal: choose 4 4,800 kcal: choose 4 4,900 kcal: choose 4
Nonstarchy vegetables	1 cup (56 g) dark green lettuce 15 raw baby carrots 1 large tomato 1/2 cup (62 g) cooked green beans 1/2 cup (78 g) cooked broccoli 1/2 cup (62 g) cooked cauliflower 1/2 cup (90 g) cooked zucchini 1 medium onion 1 bell pepper	4,400 kcal: choose 8 4,500 kcal: choose 8 4,600 kcal: choose 9 4,700 kcal: choose 9 4,800 kcal: choose 9 4,900 kcal: choose 9
Fruits	1 small apple 1 small banana 1 cup (144 g) berries 1 small orange 2 tbsp (18 g) raisins 1/2 cup (120 ml) 100% fruit juice 17 grapes 1/2 cup (122 g) unsweetened applesauce 1/2 cup (128 g) cut fresh or canned fruit, unsweetened	4,400 kcal: choose 12 4,500 kcal: choose 12 4,600 kcal: choose 12 4,700 kcal: choose 13 4,800 kcal: choose 13 4,900 kcal: choose 13
Grains and starches	1 slice bread 1/2 6-in. (15 cm) pita 1/2 English muffin 1/2 small (2 oz or 60 g) bagel 1/4 large (4 oz or 120 g) bagel 1/2 cup (121 g) cooked cereal 3/4 cup (21 g) unsweetened ready-to-eat cereal 1 4-in. (10 cm) thin pancake 1 4-in. (10 cm) square waffle 1/2 cup (93 g) cooked rice 1/2 cup (70 g) cooked pasta 1/3 cup (83 g) baked beans 1/2 cup (82 g) corn 1/4 large (3 oz or 90 g) potato 1 small dinner roll 3 graham cracker squares	4,400 kcal: choose 18 4,500 kcal: choose 18 4,600 kcal: choose 18 4,700 kcal: choose 18 4,800 kcal: choose 19 4,900 kcal: choose 20
Foods with sugar	1 energy or granola bar (~1 oz or 30 g) 1 frozen 100% fruit juice bar 1 tbsp (21 g) honey, jam, or syrup or 1 tbsp (12 g) sugar 1 cup (8 oz or 240 ml) sports drink 1/2 cup (87 g) frozen yogurt	4,400 kcal: choose 4 4,500 kcal: choose 5 4,600 kcal: choose 5 4,700 kcal: choose 5 4,800 kcal: choose 5 4,900 kcal: choose 5

Lean protein	1 oz (30 g) (very thin slice) *lean*
	  chicken
	  turkey
	  beef
	  pork
	  fish
	2 egg whites or 1/4 cup (61 g) egg substitute
		4,400 kcal: choose 12
		4,500 kcal: choose 12
		4,600 kcal: choose 12
		4,700 kcal: choose 12
		4,800 kcal: choose 12
		4,900 kcal: choose 12

Fats and oils	1 tsp (5 g) margarine 1 tbsp (15 g) reduced-fat margarine 1 tsp (5 g) oil 1 tsp (5 g) mayo 1 tbsp (14 g) reduced-fat mayo 1/2 tbsp (8 g) peanut or almond butter 1 tbsp (14 g) cream cheese 1 tbsp (16 g) salad dressing 2 tbsp (29 g) avocado 6 almonds 4 walnut halves 10 peanuts	4,400 kcal: choose 22 4,500 kcal: choose 22 4,600 kcal: choose 23 4,700 kcal: choose 24 4,800 kcal: choose 25 4,900 kcal: choose 25

Sample 4,900-Calorie One-Day Menu

Meal or snack	Amount and food	Number of choices and food group
Breakfast	1 1/2 cup (42 g) unsweetened ready-to-eat cereal	2 grains and starches
	1 small banana	1 fruits
	1 whole-grain English muffin	2 grains and starches
	5 tsp (25 g) margarine	5 fats and oils
	4 scrambled egg whites or 1/2 cup egg substitute	2 lean protein
	1 cup (150 g) chopped raw vegetables	1 nonstarchy vegetables
	8 oz (1 cup or 240 ml) orange juice	2 fruits
	8 oz (1 cup or 240 ml) skim milk	1 fat-free milk and yogurt
Lunch	1 1/2 whole-wheat pita bread	3 grains and starches
	4 oz (120 g) chicken breast	4 lean protein
	Spinach leaves, sliced tomato, and sliced cucumber	1 nonstarchy vegetables
	15 raw baby carrots	1 nonstarchy vegetables
	1 bell pepper	1 nonstarchy vegetables
	3 tbsp (42 g) reduced-fat mayo	3 fats and oils
	8 walnut halves	2 fats and oils
	1 small apple	1 fruits
	1 large orange	2 fruits
	Calorie-free beverage	
Preexercise snack	1 large banana	2 fruits
	6 squares graham crackers	2 grains and starches
	20 oz (2 1/2 cup or 600 ml) sports drink	2 1/2 foods with sugar
Postexercise snack	8 oz (1 cup or 240 ml) low fat kefir	1 fat-free milk and yogurt
	6 tbsp (48 g) raisins	3 fruits
	50 peanuts	5 fats and oils
	3 cups (84 g) unsweetened ready-to-eat cereal	4 grains and starches
	20 oz (2 1/2 cup or 600 ml) sports drink	2 1/2 foods with sugar
Dinner	6 oz (180 g) grilled salmon	6 lean protein
	1 1/2 cup (234 g) cooked broccoli	3 nonstarchy vegetables
	1 large (12 oz or 360 g) potato	4 grains and starches
	1 cup (56 g) dark green lettuce	1 nonstarchy vegetables
	1 cup (150 g) chopped raw pepper, tomato, carrot	1 nonstarchy vegetables
	12 walnut halves	3 fats and oils
	2 tbsp (32 g) salad dressing	2 fats and oils
	3 whole-wheat rolls	3 grains and starches
	5 tsp (25 g) margarine	5 fats and oils
	1 cup (256 g) cut fresh fruit	2 fruits
	16 oz (2 cups or 480 ml) skim milk	2 fat-free milk and yogurt

Building Muscle and Losing Fat

This chapter is designed for athletes who want to gain muscle mass and lose body fat simultaneously. (If your goal is only to gain muscle, turn to chapter 10. If you want only to lose fat, see chapter 11.) Many athletes have this two-pronged goal as they try to achieve a body weight and composition that is well matched to their sport and position. Body weight may increase, decrease, or stay the same, depending on how much muscle mass is gained and how much body fat is lost. Losing body fat and building muscle at the same time requires precise caloric intake. Consuming too many calories will hamper your efforts to lose body fat, but taking in too few calories will impede muscle growth.

To gain muscle and lose body fat at the same time, you must do three things:

- Consume the right number of calories
- Consume the proper amounts and proportions of protein, carbohydrate, and fat
- Engage in a program of resistance exercise without overtraining

You need to determine your baseline calories before you can begin building muscle and losing fat. If your current body weight is stable, you can use as your baseline the figures that you obtained in calculating your average daily caloric intake as explained in chapter 3. If you are currently gaining or losing weight, then you should calculate your estimated caloric need as explained in chapter 5. This estimate takes into account your physical activity level, which may be greater than usual because of additional resistance training. A large discrepancy between your current intake and your estimated caloric need suggests that you need to reconcile and fine-tune your baseline caloric estimate.

The appropriate calorie range for simultaneously building muscle and losing fat is narrow, so you need to be precise in determining how many calories you need. Therefore, you must accurately measure your current food intake and specifically record your physical activity. This level of precision will increase your accuracy in predicting your calorie needs. Nonetheless, you should evaluate your progress regularly to assess whether you are within the appropriate range and be ready to adjust your calorie level as needed.

After you have determined your baseline calories, increase the calories by the amount shown in table 12.1. You must take in sufficient calories to support resistance training and fuel muscle growth, but you want some of the calories needed to come from stored body fat. To accomplish your goals, your caloric intake must be precise. Therefore, you should periodically reassess your daily caloric intake. If you are not increasing muscle mass, increase your caloric intake by 50 to 100 kilocalories daily. If you are not losing body fat, decrease your caloric intake by 50 to 100 kilocalories daily. Continue to adjust your estimated caloric intake until you are meeting your goals.

TABLE 12.1

Calories Needed to Build Muscle and Lose Fat

Goal	Gender	Total calories
To gain muscle mass and lose body fat simultaneously	Male	Baseline kcal plus 300 kcal
	Female	Baseline kcal plus 200 kcal

Select Your Jumpstart Meal Plan

When you know how many calories you need, you are ready to choose a jumpstart meal plan for that calorie level. The plans in this chapter are simple to use and will help you get off to a good start in your effort to lose body fat while gaining muscle. By following these simple plans exactly, you can establish a pattern of eating that will help you reach your body-composition and performance goals. The plans in this chapter are easy to follow because they offer a limited number of food choices.

This simplicity, however, results from a lack of variety. A monotonous diet is difficult to follow over time and restricts the range of nutrient intake, so you should not use this plan for more than a week or two. You can expand the foods in this diet by creating a customized, personal plan using the precision meal planning system described in chapter 13. By creating a diet with a variety of your favorite foods, you will be able to follow your customized plan over the months required to meet your goals.

Each meal plan has been designed to contain the proper amount and proportions of carbohydrate, protein, and fat to support maximum muscle gain and a modest fat loss. They have been calculated to contain approximately 7 grams of carbohydrate, 1.7 grams of protein, and between 1 and 2 grams of fat per kilogram of body weight.

The meal plan includes seven food groups. Your meal plan lists the total number of choices that you can make from each group. You are free to choose whichever foods you like within each food group. To maintain the right calorie level and macronutrient balance, you need to eat foods and beverages in the quantities specified.

You can select the plan that is right for you by following these simple steps:

1. Select the correct calorie range for your needs based on table 12.1. The meal plans are provided in 500 kilocalorie increments. For example, if you need 3,700 kilocalories daily, you should use the 3,400 to 3,800 kilocalories meal plan.

2. According to your calorie level, choose the correct number of foods from each food group. For example, a 3,700-kilocalorie diet consists of two choices from the fat-free milk and yogurt group, seven choices from the nonstarchy vegetables group, and so on. When the plan requires you to choose more than one food from a group, you may select any combination to reach the total number of choices. You may choose each food listed more than once. For example, two fat-free milk and yogurt choices could be two 8-ounce (240-milliliter) glasses of fat-free milk or one 8-ounce (240-milliliter) glass of soy milk and 6 ounces (180 grams) of fat-free yogurt. Several options are available in each food group, but remember that the total number of choices for the day should not exceed or fall below the recommended level.

3. From the foods chosen, create three meals and two snacks. Eat the snacks before and after you exercise.

You can use the four sample menus as an example of how to translate the number of choices in the meal plan into meals and snacks (see chapter 13 for more information). The meals and snacks that you create may be different from these sample menus because each food group has several foods to choose from. When you divide the total choices in your meal plan into meals and snacks, remember that you should have at least three meals and two snacks each day. To build muscle, be sure to consume some carbohydrate and protein in the first hour after exercise (see chapter 6).

2,400- to 2,800-Calorie Meal Plan

Food group	Food group choices	Calorie level and number of choices
Fat-free milk and yogurt	8 oz (240 ml) fat-free or 1% milk 8 oz (240 ml) soy milk 8 oz (240 ml) low-fat kefir 6 oz (180 g) fat-free yogurt	2,400 kcal: choose 2 2,500 kcal: choose 2 2,600 kcal: choose 2 2,700 kcal: choose 2 2,800 kcal: choose 2
Nonstarchy vegetables	1 cup (56 g) dark green lettuce 15 raw baby carrots 1 large tomato 1/2 cup (62 g) cooked green beans 1/2 cup (78 g) cooked broccoli 1/2 cup (62 g) cooked cauliflower 1/2 cup (90 g) cooked zucchini 1 medium onion 1 bell pepper	2,400 kcal: choose 5 2,500 kcal: choose 5 2,600 kcal: choose 5 2,700 kcal: choose 5 2,800 kcal: choose 6
Fruits	1 small apple 1 small banana 1 cup (144 g) berries 1 small orange 2 tbsp (18 g) raisins 1/2 cup (120 ml) 100% fruit juice 17 grapes 1/2 cup (122 g) unsweetened applesauce 1/2 cup (128 g) cut fresh or canned fruit, unsweetened	2,400 kcal: choose 11 2,500 kcal: choose 11 2,600 kcal: choose 11 2,700 kcal: choose 11 2,800 kcal: choose 12
Grains and starches	1 slice bread 1/2 6-in. (15 cm) pita 1/2 English muffin 1/2 small (2 oz or 60 g) bagel 1/4 large (4 oz or 120 g) bagel 1/2 cup (121 g) cooked cereal 3/4 cup (21 g) unsweetened ready-to-eat cereal 1 4-in. (10 cm) thin pancake 1 4-in. (10 cm) square waffle 1/2 cup (93 g) cooked rice 1/2 cup (70 g) cooked pasta 1/3 cup (83 g) baked beans 1/2 cup (82 g) corn 1/4 large (3 oz or 90 g) potato 1 small dinner roll 3 graham cracker squares	2,400 kcal: choose 9 2,500 kcal: choose 9 2,600 kcal: choose 10 2,700 kcal: choose 11 2,800 kcal: choose 11
Foods with sugar	1 energy or granola bar (~1 oz or 30 g) 1 frozen 100% fruit juice bar 1 tbsp (21 g) honey, jam, or syrup or 1 tbsp (12 g) sugar 1 cup (8 oz or 240 ml) sports drink 1/2 cup (87 g) frozen yogurt	2,400 kcal: choose 0 2,500 kcal: choose 1 2,600 kcal: choose 1 2,700 kcal: choose 1 2,800 kcal: choose 1

Lean protein	1 oz (30 g) (very thin slice) *lean*
	   chicken
	   turkey
	   beef
	   pork
	   fish
	2 egg whites or 1/4 cup (61 g) egg substitute
		2,400 kcal: choose 5
		2,500 kcal: choose 5
		2,600 kcal: choose 5
		2,700 kcal: choose 5
		2,800 kcal: choose 5

Fats and oils	1 tsp (5 g) margarine 1 tbsp (15 g) reduced-fat margarine 1 tsp (5 g) oil 1 tsp (5 g) mayo 1 tbsp (14 g) reduced-fat mayo 1/2 tbsp (8 g) peanut or almond butter 1 tbsp (14 g) cream cheese 1 tbsp (16 g) salad dressing 2 tbsp (29 g) avocado 6 almonds 4 walnut halves 10 peanuts	2,400 kcal: choose 12 2,500 kcal: choose 12 2,600 kcal: choose 12 2,700 kcal: choose 13 2,800 kcal: choose 14

Sample 2,400-Calorie One-Day Menu

Meal or snack	Amount and food	Number of choices and food group
Breakfast	1/2 cup (121 g) cooked oatmeal	1 grains and starches
	2 tbsp (18 g) raisins	1 fruits
	4 walnut halves	1 fats and oils
	1 whole-wheat English muffin	2 grains and starches
	1 tbsp (16 g) peanut butter	2 fats and oils
	4 oz (1/2 cup, or 120 ml) orange juice	1 fruits
	8 oz (1 cup or 240 ml) skim milk	1 fat-free milk and yogurt
Lunch	2 slices whole-grain rye bread	2 grains and starches
	2 oz (60 g) tuna, water packed	2 lean protein
	Lettuce, tomato, and onion slices	1 nonstarchy vegetables
	2 tbsp (28 g) reduced-fat mayo	2 fats and oils
	1 cup (56 g) dark green lettuce	1 nonstarchy vegetables
	1 cup (150 g) chopped raw tomato, onion, carrot	1 nonstarchy vegetables
	1 tbsp (16 g) salad dressing	1 fats and oils
	8 oz (1 cup or 240 ml) 100% fruit juice	2 fruits
	1 cup (144 g) strawberries	1 fruits
Preexercise snack	1 large banana	2 fruits
Postexercise snack	8 oz (1 cup or 240 ml) low-fat kefir	1 fat-free milk and yogurt
	4 tbsp (36 g) raisins	2 fruits
	3/4 cup (21 g) Cheerios	1 grains and starches
	20 peanuts, salted	2 fats and oils
	Water to replace fluid lost during exercise	
Dinner	3 oz (90 g) very lean baked ham	3 lean protein
	1/2 large (6 oz or 180 g) potato	2 grains and starches
	1/2 cup (82 g) corn	1 grains and starches
	1 cup (56 g) dark green lettuce	1 nonstarchy vegetables
	1 large tomato	1 nonstarchy vegetables
	2 tsp (10 g) margarine	2 fats and oils
	2 tbsp (32 g) salad dressing	2 fats and oils
	1 cup (244 g) unsweetened applesauce	2 fruits
	Calorie-free beverage	

2,900- to 3,300-Calorie Meal Plan

Food group	Food group choices	Calorie level and number of choices
Fat-free milk and yogurt	8 oz (240 ml) fat-free or 1% milk 8 oz (240 ml) soy milk 8 oz (240 ml) low-fat kefir 6 oz (180 g) fat-free yogurt	2,900 kcal: choose 2 3,000 kcal: choose 2 3,100 kcal: choose 2 3,200 kcal: choose 2 3,300 kcal: choose 2
Nonstarchy vegetables	1 cup (56 g) dark green lettuce 15 raw baby carrots 1 large tomato 1/2 cup (62 g) cooked green beans 1/2 cup (78 g) cooked broccoli 1/2 cup (62 g) cooked cauliflower 1/2 cup (90 g) cooked zucchini 1 medium onion 1 bell pepper	2,900 kcal: choose 6 3,000 kcal: choose 6 3,100 kcal: choose 7 3,200 kcal: choose 7 3,300 kcal: choose 7
Fruits	1 small apple 1 small banana 1 cup (144 g) berries 1 small orange 2 tbsp (18 g) raisins 1/2 cup (120 ml) 100% fruit juice 17 grapes 1/2 cup (122 g) unsweetened applesauce 1/2 cup (128 g) cut fresh or canned fruit, unsweetened	2,900 kcal: choose 12 3,000 kcal: choose 12 3,100 kcal: choose 13 3,200 kcal: choose 13 3,300 kcal: choose 13
Grains and starches	1 slice bread 1/2 6-in. (15 cm) pita 1/2 English muffin 1/2 small (2 oz or 60 g) bagel 1/4 large (4 oz or 120 g) bagel 1/2 cup (121 g) cooked cereal 3/4 cup (21 g) unsweetened ready-to-eat cereal 1 4-in. (10 cm) thin pancake 1 4-in. (10 cm) square waffle 1/2 cup (93 g) cooked rice 1/2 cup (70 g) cooked pasta 1/3 cup (83 g) baked beans 1/2 cup (82 g) corn 1/4 large (3 oz or 90 g) potato 1 small dinner roll 3 graham cracker squares	2,900 kcal: choose 11 3,000 kcal: choose 12 3,100 kcal: choose 12 3,200 kcal: choose 13 3,300 kcal: choose 13
Foods with sugar	1 energy or granola bar (~1 oz or 30 g) 1 frozen 100% fruit juice bar 1 tbsp (21 g) honey, jam, or syrup or 1 tbsp (12 g) sugar 1 cup (8 oz or 240 ml) sports drink 1/2 cup (87 g) frozen yogurt	2,900 kcal: choose 2 3,000 kcal: choose 2 3,100 kcal: choose 2 3,200 kcal: choose 2 3,300 kcal: choose 3

Lean protein	1 oz (30 g) (very thin slice) *lean*
	    chicken
	    turkey
	    beef
	    pork
	    fish
	2 egg whites or 1/4 cup (61 g) egg substitute
		2,900 kcal: choose 7
		3,000 kcal: choose 7
		3,100 kcal: choose 7
		3,200 kcal: choose 7
		3,300 kcal: choose 8

Fats and oils	1 tsp (5 g) margarine 1 tbsp (15 g) reduced-fat margarine 1 tsp (5 g) oil 1 tsp (5 g) mayo 1 tbsp (14 g) reduced-fat mayo 1/2 tbsp (8 g) peanut or almond butter 1 tbsp (14 g) cream cheese 1 tbsp (16 g) salad dressing 2 tbsp (29 g) avocado 6 almonds 4 walnut halves 10 peanuts	2,900 kcal: choose 12 3,000 kcal: choose 12 3,100 kcal: choose 13 3,200 kcal: choose 13 3,300 kcal: choose 13

3,400- to 3,800-Calorie Meal Plan

Food group	Food group choices	Calorie level and number of choices
Fat-free milk and yogurt	8 oz (240 ml) fat-free or 1% milk 8 oz (240 ml) soy milk 8 oz (240 ml) low-fat kefir 6 oz (180 g) fat-free yogurt	3,400 kcal: choose 2 3,500 kcal: choose 2 3,600 kcal: choose 2 3,700 kcal: choose 2 3,800 kcal: choose 2
Nonstarchy vegetables	1 cup (56 g) dark green lettuce 15 raw baby carrots 1 large tomato 1/2 cup (62 g) cooked green beans 1/2 cup (78 g) cooked broccoli 1/2 cup (62 g) cooked cauliflower 1/2 cup (90 g) cooked zucchini 1 medium onion 1 bell pepper	3,400 kcal: choose 7 3,500 kcal: choose 7 3,600 kcal: choose 7 3,700 kcal: choose 7 3,800 kcal: choose 7
Fruits	1 small apple 1 small banana 1 cup (144 g) berries 1 small orange 2 tbsp (18 g) raisins 1/2 cup (120 ml) 100% fruit juice 17 grapes 1/2 cup (122 g) unsweetened applesauce 1/2 cup (128 g) cut fresh or canned fruit, unsweetened	3,400 kcal: choose 13 3,500 kcal: choose 13 3,600 kcal: choose 13 3,700 kcal: choose 13 3,800 kcal: choose 14
Grains and starches	1 slice bread 1/2 6-in. (15 cm) pita 1/2 English muffin 1/2 small (2 oz or 60 g) bagel 1/4 large (4 oz or 120 g) bagel 1/2 cup (121 g) cooked cereal 3/4 cup (21 g) unsweetened ready-to-eat cereal 1 4-in. (10 cm) thin pancake 1 4-in. (10 cm) square waffle 1/2 cup (93 g) cooked rice 1/2 cup (70 g) cooked pasta 1/3 cup (83 g) baked beans 1/2 cup (82 g) corn 1/4 large (3 oz or 90 g) potato 1 small dinner roll 3 graham cracker squares	3,400 kcal: choose 14 3,500 kcal: choose 15 3,600 kcal: choose 16 3,700 kcal: choose 17 3,800 kcal: choose 17
Foods with sugar	1 energy or granola bar (~1 oz or 30 g) 1 frozen 100% fruit juice bar 1 tbsp (21 g) honey, jam, or syrup or 1 tbsp (12 g) sugar 1 cup (8 oz or 240 ml) sports drink 1/2 cup (87 g) frozen yogurt	3,400 kcal: choose 3 3,500 kcal: choose 3 3,600 kcal: choose 3 3,700 kcal: choose 3 3,800 kcal: choose 3

Lean protein	1 oz (30 g) (very thin slice) *lean*
	    chicken
	    turkey
	    beef
	    pork
	    fish
	2 egg whites or 1/4 cup (61 g) egg substitute
		3,400 kcal: choose 8
		3,500 kcal: choose 8
		3,600 kcal: choose 8
		3,700 kcal: choose 8
		3,800 kcal: choose 9

Fats and oils	1 tsp (5 g) margarine 1 tbsp (15 g) reduced-fat margarine 1 tsp (5 g) oil 1 tsp (5 g) mayo 1 tbsp (14 g) reduced-fat mayo 1/2 tbsp (8 g) peanut or almond butter 1 tbsp (14 g) cream cheese 1 tbsp (16 g) salad dressing 2 tbsp (29 g) avocado 6 almonds 4 walnut halves 10 peanuts	3,400 kcal: choose 14 3,500 kcal: choose 14 3,600 kcal: choose 15 3,700 kcal: choose 16 3,800 kcal: choose 16

Sample 3,400-Calorie One-Day Menu

Meal or snack	Amount and food	Number of choices and food group
Breakfast	1 cup (242 g) cooked oatmeal	2 grains and starches
	4 tbsp (36 g) raisins	2 fruits
	6 almonds	1 fats and oils
	1 whole-wheat English muffin	2 grains and starches
	1 1/2 tbsp (24 g) peanut butter	3 fats and oils
	8 oz (1 cup or 240 ml) orange juice	2 fruits
	8 oz (1 cup or 240 ml) fat-free milk	1 fat-free milk and yogurt
Lunch	3 slices whole-grain rye bread	3 grains and starches
	4 oz (120 g) tuna, water packed	4 lean protein
	Lettuce, tomato, and onion slices	1 nonstarchy vegetables
	1 tbsp (14 g) reduced-fat mayo	1 fats and oils
	1 cup (56 g) dark green lettuce	1 nonstarchy vegetables
	1 cup (150 g) chopped raw tomato, onion, carrot	1 nonstarchy vegetables
	2 tbsp (32 g) salad dressing	2 fats and oils
	8 oz (1 cup or 240 ml) 100% fruit juice	2 fruits
	1 cup (144 g) strawberries	1 fruits
Preexercise snack	1 large banana	2 fruits
	3 squares graham crackers	1 grains and starches
	8 oz (1 cup or 240 ml) sports drink	1 foods with sugar
Postexercise snack	8 oz (1 cup or 240 ml) low-fat kefir	1 fat-free milk and yogurt
	1 small apple	1 fruits
	2 tbsp (18 g) raisins	1 fruits
	1 1/2 cups (42 g) Cheerios	2 grains and starches
	30 peanuts	3 fats and oils
	16 oz (2 cups, or 480 ml) sports drink	2 foods with sugar
Dinner	4 oz (120 g) baked very lean ham	4 lean protein
	1 large (12 oz or 360 g) potato	4 grains and starches
	1 cup (124 g) green beans	2 nonstarchy vegetables
	1 cup (56 g) dark green lettuce	1 nonstarchy vegetables
	1 large tomato	1 nonstarchy vegetables
	2 tsp (10 g) margarine	2 fats and oils
	2 tbsp (32 g) salad dressing	2 fats and oils
	1 cup (244 g) unsweetened applesauce	2 fruits
	Calorie-free beverage	

3,900- to 4,300-Calorie Meal Plan

Food group	Food group choices	Calorie level and number of choices
Fat-free milk and yogurt	8 oz (240 ml) fat-free or 1% milk 8 oz (240 ml) soy milk 8 oz (240 ml) low-fat kefir 6 oz (180 g) fat-free yogurt	3,900 kcal: choose 2 4,000 kcal: choose 3 4,100 kcal: choose 3 4,200 kcal: choose 3 4,300 kcal: choose 3
Nonstarchy vegetables	1 cup (56 g) dark green lettuce 15 raw baby carrots 1 large tomato 1/2 cup (62 g) cooked green beans 1/2 cup (78 g) cooked broccoli 1/2 cup (62 g) cooked cauliflower 1/2 cup (90 g) cooked zucchini 1 medium onion 1 bell pepper	3,900 kcal: choose 7 4,000 kcal: choose 7 4,100 kcal: choose 7 4,200 kcal: choose 7 4,300 kcal: choose 7
Fruits	1 small apple 1 small banana 1 cup (144 g) berries 1 small orange 2 tbsp (18 g) raisins 1/2 cup (120 ml) 100% fruit juice 17 grapes 1/2 cup (122 g) unsweetened applesauce 1/2 cup (128 g) cut fresh or canned fruit, unsweetened	3,900 kcal: choose 14 4,000 kcal: choose 13 4,100 kcal: choose 14 4,200 kcal: choose 14 4,300 kcal: choose 14
Grains and starches	1 slice bread 1/2 6-in. (15 cm) pita 1/2 English muffin 1/2 small (2 oz or 60 g) bagel 1/4 large (4 oz or 120 g) bagel 1/2 cup (121 g) cooked cereal 3/4 cup (21 g) unsweetened ready-to-eat cereal 1 4-in. (10 cm) thin pancake 1 4-in. (10 cm) square waffle 1/2 cup (93 g) cooked rice 1/2 cup (70 g) cooked pasta 1/3 cup (83 g) baked beans 1/2 cup (82 g) corn 1/4 large (3 oz or 90 g) potato 1 small dinner roll 3 graham cracker squares	3,900 kcal: choose 17 4,000 kcal: choose 18 4,100 kcal: choose 18 4,200 kcal: choose 19 4,300 kcal: choose 20
Foods with sugar	1 energy or granola bar (~1 oz or 30 g) 1 frozen 100% fruit juice bar 1 tbsp (21 g) honey, jam, or syrup or 1 tbsp (12 g) sugar 1 cup (8 oz or 240 ml) sports drink 1/2 cup (87 g) frozen yogurt	3,900 kcal: choose 4 4,000 kcal: choose 4 4,100 kcal: choose 4 4,200 kcal: choose 4 4,300 kcal: choose 4

Lean protein	1 oz (30 g) (very thin slice) *lean*
	    chicken
	    turkey
	    beef
	    pork
	    fish
	2 egg whites or 1/4 cup (61 g) egg substitute
		3,900 kcal: choose 9
		4,000 kcal: choose 8
		4,100 kcal: choose 9
		4,200 kcal: choose 9
		4,300 kcal: choose 9

Fats and oils	1 tsp (5 g) margarine 1 tbsp (15 g) reduced-fat margarine 1 tsp (5 g) oil 1 tsp (5 g) mayo 1 tbsp (14 g) reduced-fat mayo 1/2 tbsp (8 g) peanut or almond butter 1 tbsp (14 g) cream cheese 1 tbsp (16 g) salad dressing 2 tbsp (29 g) avocado 6 almonds 4 walnut halves 10 peanuts	3,900 kcal: choose 16 4,000 kcal: choose 17 4,100 kcal: choose 17 4,200 kcal: choose 18 4,300 kcal: choose 18

4,400- to 4,800-Calorie Meal Plan

Food group	Food group choices	Calorie level and number of choices
Fat-free milk and yogurt	8 oz (240 ml) fat-free or 1% milk 8 oz (240 ml) soy milk 8 oz (240 ml) low-fat kefir 6 oz (180 g) fat-free yogurt	4,400 kcal: choose 3 4,500 kcal: choose 3 4,600 kcal: choose 3 4,700 kcal: choose 3 4,800 kcal: choose 3
Nonstarchy vegetables	1 cup (56 g) dark green lettuce 15 raw baby carrots 1 large tomato 1/2 cup (62 g) cooked green beans 1/2 cup (78 g) cooked broccoli 1/2 cup (62 g) cooked cauliflower 1/2 cup (90 g) cooked zucchini 1 medium onion 1 bell pepper	4,400 kcal: choose 7 4,500 kcal: choose 7 4,600 kcal: choose 7 4,700 kcal: choose 7 4,800 kcal: choose 7
Fruits	1 small apple 1 small banana 1 cup (144 g) berries 1 small orange 2 tbsp (18 g) raisins 1/2 cup (120 ml) 100% fruit juice 17 grapes 1/2 cup (122 g) unsweetened applesauce 1/2 cup (128 g) cut fresh or canned fruit, unsweetened	4,400 kcal: choose 14 4,500 kcal: choose 15 4,600 kcal: choose 15 4,700 kcal: choose 15 4,800 kcal: choose 15
Grains and starches	1 slice bread 1/2 6-in. (15 cm) pita 1/2 English muffin 1/2 small (2 oz or 60 g) bagel 1/4 large (4 oz or 120 g) bagel 1/2 cup (121 g) cooked cereal 3/4 cup (21 g) unsweetened ready-to-eat cereal 1 4-in. (10 cm) thin pancake 1 4-in. (10 cm) square waffle 1/2 cup (93 g) cooked rice 1/2 cup (70 g) cooked pasta 1/3 cup (83 g) baked beans 1/2 cup (82 g) corn 1/4 large (3 oz or 90 g) potato 1 small dinner roll 3 graham cracker squares	4,400 kcal: choose 20 4,500 kcal: choose 20 4,600 kcal: choose 21 4,700 kcal: choose 21 4,800 kcal: choose 22
Foods with sugar	1 energy or granola bar (~1 oz or 30 g) 1 frozen 100% fruit juice bar 1 tbsp (21 g) honey, jam, or syrup or 1 tbsp (12 g) sugar 1 cup (8 oz or 240 ml) sports drink 1/2 cup (87 g) frozen yogurt	4,400 kcal: choose 5 4,500 kcal: choose 5 4,600 kcal: choose 5 4,700 kcal: choose 6 4,800 kcal: choose 6

Lean protein	1 oz (30 g) (very thin slice) *lean*
	   chicken
	   turkey
	   beef
	   pork
	   fish
	2 egg whites or 1/4 cup (61 g) egg substitute
		4,400 kcal: choose 9
		4,500 kcal: choose 10
		4,600 kcal: choose 10
		4,700 kcal: choose 11
		4,800 kcal: choose 11

Fats and oils	1 tsp (5 g) margarine 1 tbsp (15 g) reduced-fat margarine 1 tsp (5 g) oil 1 tsp (5 g) mayo 1 tbsp (14 g) reduced-fat mayo 1/2 tbsp (8 g) peanut or almond butter 1 tbsp (14 g) cream cheese 1 tbsp (16 g) salad dressing 2 tbsp (29 g) avocado 6 almonds 4 walnut halves 10 peanuts	4,400 kcal: choose 19 4,500 kcal: choose 19 4,600 kcal: choose 19 4,700 kcal: choose 19 4,800 kcal: choose 20

Sample 4,400-Calorie One-Day Menu

Meal or snack	Amount and food	Number of choices and food group
Breakfast	1 1/2 cup (363 g) cooked oatmeal	3 grains and starches
	4 tbsp (36 g) raisins	2 fruits
	1 tbsp (12 g) sugar	1 foods with sugar
	12 almonds	2 fats and oils
	1 whole-wheat English muffin	2 grains and starches
	2 tbsp (32 g) peanut butter	4 fats and oils
	8 oz (1 cup or 240 ml) orange juice	2 fruits
	8 oz (1 cup or 240 ml) fat-free milk	1 fat-free milk and yogurt
Lunch	4 slices whole-grain rye bread	4 grains and starches
	4 oz (120 g) tuna, water packed	4 lean protein
	Lettuce, tomato, and onion	1 nonstarchy vegetables
	4 tbsp (56 g) reduced-fat mayo	4 fats and oils
	1 cup (56 g) dark green lettuce	1 nonstarchy vegetables
	1 cup (150 g) chopped raw tomato, onion, carrot	1 nonstarchy vegetables
	2 tbsp (32 g) salad dressing	2 fats and oils
	8 oz (1 cup or 240 ml) 100% fruit juice	2 fruits
	1 cup (144 g) strawberries	1 fruits
Preexercise snack	1 large banana	2 fruits
	6 squares graham crackers	2 grains and starches
	16 oz (2 cups or 480 ml) sports drink	2 foods with sugar
Postexercise snack	8 oz (1 cup or 240 ml) low-fat kefir	1 fat-free milk and yogurt
	1 small apple	1 fruits
	4 tbsp (36 g) raisins	2 fruits
	2 1/4 cups (63 g) Cheerios	3 grains and starches
	30 peanuts	3 fats and oils
	16 oz (2 cups or 480 ml) sports drink	2 foods with sugar
Dinner	5 oz (150 g) very lean baked ham	5 lean protein
	1 large (12 oz or 360 g) potato	4 grains and starches
	1 cup (164 g) corn	2 grains and starches
	1 cup (124 g) green beans	2 nonstarchy vegetables
	1 cup (56 g) dark green lettuce	1 nonstarchy vegetables
	1 large tomato	1 nonstarchy vegetables
	2 tsp (10 g) margarine	2 fats and oils
	2 tbsp (32 g) salad dressing	2 fats and oils
	1 cup (244 g) unsweetened applesauce	2 fruits
	8 oz (1 cup or 240 ml) fat-free milk	1 fat-free milk and yogurt

4,900- to 5,300-Calorie Meal Plan

Food group	Food group choices	Calorie level and number of choices
Fat-free milk and yogurt	8 oz (240 ml) fat-free or 1% milk 8 oz (240 ml) soy milk 8 oz (240 ml) low-fat kefir 6 oz (180 g) fat-free yogurt	4,900 kcal: choose 3 5,000 kcal: choose 4 5,100 kcal: choose 4 5,200 kcal: choose 4 5,300 kcal: choose 4
Nonstarchy vegetables	1 cup (56 g) dark green lettuce 15 raw baby carrots 1 large tomato 1/2 cup (62 g) cooked green beans 1/2 cup (78 g) cooked broccoli 1/2 cup (62 g) cooked cauliflower 1/2 cup (90 g) cooked zucchini 1 medium onion 1 bell pepper	4,900 kcal: choose 7 5,000 kcal: choose 7 5,100 kcal: choose 7 5,200 kcal: choose 7 5,300 kcal: choose 7
Fruits	1 small apple 1 small banana 1 cup (144 g) berries 1 small orange 2 tbsp (18 g) raisins 1/2 cup (120 ml) 100% fruit juice 17 grapes 1/2 cup (122 g) unsweetened applesauce 1/2 cup (128 g) cut fresh or canned fruit, unsweetened	4,900 kcal: choose 15 5,000 kcal: choose 15 5,100 kcal: choose 15 5,200 kcal: choose 15 5,300 kcal: choose 15
Grains and starches	1 slice bread 1/2 6-in. (15 cm) pita 1/2 English muffin 1/2 small (2 oz or 60 g) bagel 1/4 large(4 oz or 120 g) bagel 1/2 cup (121 g) cooked cereal 3/4 cup (21 g) unsweetened ready-to-eat cereal 1 4-in. (10 cm) thin pancake 1 4-in. (10 cm) square waffle 1/2 cup (93 g) cooked rice 1/2 cup (70 g) cooked pasta 1/3 cup (83 g) baked beans 1/2 cup (82 g) corn 1/4 large (3 oz or 90 g) potato 1 small dinner roll 3 graham cracker squares	4,900 kcal: choose 23 5,000 kcal: choose 23 5,100 kcal: choose 23 5,200 kcal: choose 24 5,300 kcal: choose 25
Foods with sugar	1 energy or granola bar (~1 oz or 30 g) 1 frozen 100% fruit juice bar 1 tbsp (21 g) honey, jam, or syrup or 1 tbsp (12 g) sugar 1 cup (8 oz or 240 ml) sports drink 1/2 cup (87 g) frozen yogurt	4,900 kcal: choose 6 5,000 kcal: choose 6 5,100 kcal: choose 7 5,200 kcal: choose 7 5,300 kcal: choose 7

Lean protein	1 oz (30 g) (very thin slice) *lean*
	   chicken
	   turkey
	   beef
	   pork
	   fish
	2 egg whites or 1/4 cup (61 g) egg substitute
		4,900 kcal: choose 11
		5,000 kcal: choose 11
		5,100 kcal: choose 11
		5,200 kcal: choose 11
		5,300 kcal: choose 11

Fats and oils	1 tsp (5 g) margarine 1 tbsp (15 g) reduced-fat margarine 1 tsp (5 g) oil 1 tsp (5 g) mayo 1 tbsp (14 g) reduced-fat mayo 1/2 tbsp (8 g) peanut or almond butter 1 tbsp (14 g) cream cheese 1 tbsp (16 g) salad dressing 2 tbsp (29 g) avocado 6 almonds 4 walnut halves 10 peanuts	4,900 kcal: choose 20 5,000 kcal: choose 21 5,100 kcal: choose 22 5,200 kcal: choose 22 5,300 kcal: choose 23

5,400- to 5,900-Calorie Meal Plan

Food group	Food group choices	Calorie level and number of choices
Fat-free milk and yogurt	8 oz (240 ml) fat-free or 1% milk 8 oz (240 ml) soy milk 8 oz (240 ml) low-fat kefir 6 oz (180 g) fat-free yogurt	5,400 kcal: choose 4 5,500 kcal: choose 4 5,600 kcal: choose 5 5,700 kcal: choose 5 5,800 kcal: choose 5 5,900 kcal: choose 5
Nonstarchy vegetables	1 cup (56 g) dark green lettuce 15 raw baby carrots 1 large tomato 1/2 cup (62 g) cooked green beans 1/2 cup (78 g) cooked broccoli 1/2 cup (62 g) cooked cauliflower 1/2 cup (90 g) cooked zucchini 1 medium onion 1 bell pepper	5,400 kcal: choose 7 5,500 kcal: choose 7 5,600 kcal: choose 7 5,700 kcal: choose 7 5,800 kcal: choose 7 5,900 kcal: choose 7
Fruits	1 small apple 1 small banana 1 cup (144 g) berries 1 small orange 2 tbsp (18 g) raisins 1/2 cup (120 ml) 100% fruit juice 17 grapes 1/2 cup (122 g) unsweetened applesauce 1/2 cup (128 g) cut fresh or canned fruit, unsweetened	5,400 kcal: choose 15 5,500 kcal: choose 16 5,600 kcal: choose 16 5,700 kcal: choose 16 5,800 kcal: choose 16 5,900 kcal: choose 17
Grains and starches	1 slice bread 1/2 6-in. (15 cm) pita 1/2 English muffin 1/2 small (2 oz or 60 g) bagel 1/4 large (4 oz or 120 g) bagel 1/2 cup (121 g) cooked cereal 3/4 cup (21 g) unsweetened ready-to-eat cereal 1 4-in. (10 cm) thin pancake 1 4-in. (10 cm) square waffle 1/2 cup (93 g) cooked rice 1/2 cup (70 g) cooked pasta 1/3 cup (83 g) baked beans 1/2 cup (82 g) corn 1/4 large (3 oz or 90 g) potato 1 small dinner roll 3 graham cracker squares	5,400 kcal: choose 25 5,500 kcal: choose 25 5,600 kcal: choose 25 5,700 kcal: choose 25 5,800 kcal: choose 25 5,900 kcal: choose 25
Foods with sugar	1 energy or granola bar (~1 oz or 30 g) 1 frozen 100% fruit juice bar 1 tbsp (21 g) honey, jam, or syrup or 1 tbsp (12 g) sugar 1 cup (8 oz or 240 ml) sports drink 1/2 cup (87 g) frozen yogurt	5,400 kcal: choose 8 5,500 kcal: choose 8 5,600 kcal: choose 8 5,700 kcal: choose 9 5,800 kcal: choose 10 5,900 kcal: choose 10

Lean protein	1 oz (30 g) (very thin slice) *lean*
	    chicken
	    turkey
	    beef
	    pork
	    fish
	2 egg whites or 1/4 cup (61 g) egg substitute
		5,400 kcal: choose 11
		5,500 kcal: choose 12
		5,600 kcal: choose 12
		5,700 kcal: choose 12
		5,800 kcal: choose 13
		5,900 kcal: choose 13

Fats and oils	1 tsp (5 g) margarine 1 tbsp (15 g) reduced-fat margarine 1 tsp (5 g) oil 1 tsp (5 g) mayo 1 tbsp (14 g) reduced-fat mayo 1/2 tbsp (8 g) peanut or almond butter 1 tbsp (14 g) cream cheese 1 tbsp (16 g) salad dressing 2 tbsp (29 g) avocado 6 almonds 4 walnut halves 10 peanuts	5,400 kcal: choose 23 5,500 kcal: choose 23 5,600 kcal: choose 24 5,700 kcal: choose 24 5,800 kcal: choose 24 5,900 kcal: choose 24

Sample 5,400-Calorie One-Day Menu

Meal or snack	Amount and food	Number of choices and food group
Breakfast	1 1/2 cup (363 g) cooked oatmeal	3 grains and starches
	4 tbsp (36 g) raisins	2 fruits
	1 tbsp (12 g) sugar	1 foods with sugar
	12 almonds	2 fats and oils
	1 whole-wheat English muffin	2 grains and starches
	2 tbsp (32 g) peanut butter	4 fats and oils
	8 oz (1 cup or 240 ml) orange juice	2 fruits
	8 oz (1 cup or 240 ml) fat-free milk	1 fat-free milk and yogurt
Lunch	1 large (4 oz or 120 g) whole-wheat bagel	4 grains and starches
	5 oz (150 g) tuna, water packed	5 lean protein
	Lettuce, tomato, and onion slices	1 nonstarchy vegetables
	4 tbsp (56 g) reduced-fat mayo	4 fats and oils
	1 cup (140 g) cooked pasta	2 grains and starches
	1 cup (56 g) dark green lettuce	1 nonstarchy vegetables
	1 cup (150 g) chopped raw tomato, onion, carrot	1 nonstarchy vegetables
	2 tbsp (32 g) salad dressing	2 fats and oils
	8 oz (1 cup or 240 ml) 100% fruit juice	2 fruits
	1 cup (144 g) strawberries	1 fruits
	1 cup (174 g) frozen yogurt	2 foods with sugar
Preexercise snack	1 large banana	2 fruits
	6 squares graham crackers	2 grains and starches
	20 oz (2 1/2 cups or 600 ml) sports drink	2 1/2 foods with sugar
Postexercise snack	8 oz (1 cup or 240 ml) low-fat kefir	1 fat-free milk and yogurt
	1 small apple	1 fruit
	4 tbsp (36 g) raisins	2 fruits
	3 cups (84 g) Cheerios	4 grains and starches
	40 peanuts	4 fats and oils
	20 oz (2 1/2 cups or 600 ml) sports drink	2 1/2 foods with sugar
Dinner	6 oz (180 g) baked very lean ham	6 lean protein
	1 large (12 oz or 360 g) potato	4 grains and starches
	2/3 cup (166 g) baked beans	2 grains and starches
	1 cup (124 g) green beans	2 nonstarchy vegetables
	1 cup (56 g) dark green lettuce	1 nonstarchy vegetables
	1 large tomato	1 nonstarchy vegetables
	5 tsp (25 g) margarine	5 fats and oils
	2 tbsp (32 g) oil-based salad dressing	2 fats and oils
	2 whole-wheat rolls	2 grains and starches
	1 1/2 cup (366 g) unsweetened applesauce	3 fruits
	16 oz (2 cups or 480 ml) fat-free milk	2 fat-free milk and yogurt

Precision Meal Planning System

Now that you have used a jumpstart meal plan to initiate your nutrition plan, you are ready to move on to the full precision meal planning system. This system is based on the three energy-producing macronutrients: carbohydrate, protein, and fat. Foods are grouped into these three main categories according to their predominant energy-producing macronutrient. You can consume each macronutrient by choosing foods from specific food groups. The lean protein food group provides protein, and the fats and oils food group provides fat. Carbohydrate can be found in five food groups: fat-free milk and yogurt, nonstarchy vegetables, fruits, grains and starches, and foods with sugar.

For each food group we provide a list of foods that have similar nutrient profiles when measured in precise amounts called exchanges. Foods within a food group have the same energy-producing nutrient profile. Therefore, each exchange within a food group contains approximately the same amount of calories and macronutrients. You may trade or swap one food for another within a food group according to your preference, in the amounts specified as one exchange. Table 13.1 shows the three main categories of macronutrients, the food groups, and the nutrient profile of one exchange.

The number of calories that you need either to build muscle or to lose body fat determines the number of exchanges from each food group in your meal plan. The jumpstart meal plan that you chose from chapter 10, 11, or 12 specifies your calorie level and the number of exchanges that you need from each food group. The precision meal planning system also provides the right distribution of carbohydrate, protein, and fat, but it gives you many more options than the jumpstart meal plan did.

You can now create a personalized meal pattern that forms the basis of daily meals and snacks. The meal pattern that you develop distributes your exchanges throughout the day, laying out the number of meals and snacks that you eat each day. This individualized long-term nutrition strategy will help you stay on target toward reaching your goals, and it will supply all the nutrients that your body requires.

TABLE 13.1

Precision Meal Planning System at a Glance

| Macronutrients | Food group | Nutrient profile of one exchange | | | Calories (kcal) |
		Carbohydrate (g)	Protein (g)	Fat (g)	
Carbohydrate	Fat-free milk and yogurt	12	8	0–3	100
	Nonstarchy vegetables	5	2		25
	Fruits	15			60
	Grains and starches	15	0–3	0–1	80
	Foods with sugar	15	Varies	Varies	Varies
Protein	Lean protein		7	0–3	45
Fat	Fats and oils			5	45

Precision Meal Planning Food Lists

The precision meal planning food lists on pages 220 through 233 provide information that will help you consume the right amount of a wide variety of foods so that you obtain the proper amount of macronutrients and number of calories every day. These lists are expanded versions of the abbreviated food lists that formed the basis of your jumpstart meal plan. The lists let you broaden the variety and increase the flexibility of your menus. For each of the seven food groups, you can choose from the list of foods provided. At each meal you follow a pattern that specifies how many exchanges you need from each food group. When selecting foods within the food groups, be sure to note the precise measurement for one exchange.

Fat-Free Milk and Yogurt.   The foods on this list (p. 220) are different types of milk (for example, fat-free, skim, soy) or yogurt or kefir. The measurement for one exchange of fluid milk is usually 1 cup (240 milliliters), but it is less for yogurt.

Nonstarchy Vegetables.   Most vegetables are found on this list (p. 221), but there are several exceptions. Starchy vegetables contain a greater amount of carbohydrate and protein than nonstarchy vegetables do. The starchy vegetables appear in the grains and starches list because they more closely match the nutrient profile of those foods. The measurement that provides one exchange for nonstarchy vegetables is usually 1 cup (~150 grams) if raw or 1/2 cup (~75 grams) if cooked.

Fruits.   Fruits and juices are on this list (p. 222). The measurement for one exchange varies considerably.

Grains and Starches. This list (p. 224) contains many foods including bread, dry cereal, cooked cereal, rice and other grains, pasta, and the starchy vegetables such as potatoes, corn, and green peas. The measurement that provides one exchange varies considerably among the different foods.

Foods With Sugar. Included on this list (p. 227) are sports beverages, energy and sports bars, and other foods that contain sugar. The measurement for one exchange varies and depends on the carbohydrate content of the food.

Lean Protein. This list (p. 230) includes lean protein foods such as meat, poultry, and fish. The measurement that provides one exchange is 1 ounce (30 grams). Other lean protein foods such as egg whites and low-fat cottage cheese have various measurements that equal one exchange. Some protein-rich foods are high in fat. When you choose these foods, you need to count the additional fat as part of your daily fats and oils allotment.

Fats and Oils. Included in this group (p. 232) are butter, margarine, mayonnaise, salad dressing, and oil. The measurement for one exchange is 1 teaspoon (5 grams). The list includes foods that may not obviously belong in this group, such as nuts, avocado, and olives. The measurement of foods on the fats and oils list varies, but all the serving sizes are small.

Although all the foods in each list have approximately the same number of calories and similar proportions of carbohydrate, protein, and fat, they do not have the same vitamin and mineral content. For example, iceberg lettuce and broccoli are on the same list, but broccoli has many more nutrients than the iceberg lettuce does. Similarly, apples and oranges are both on the fruit list, but oranges have much more vitamin C than apples do. Eat a variety of foods to ensure that you have enough vitamins and minerals.

Because you may not always be able to prepare foods at home, you should know that fast-food restaurants offer selections that contain foods from several of the food lists. To help you make selections wisely, we have calculated how many exchanges some of the more popular items available at fast-food restaurants provide. You will find fast foods on page \bb\ in appendix B. You may also have questions about some of the many products that are specially formulated for athletes, such as meal replacement drinks and protein powders. The nutrient profiles of these products do not fall neatly into one food list, so we have used the ingredient list and nutrient composition of each product to calculate the exchange equivalents. See the food list of products formulated for athletes on page 244 in appendix B.

Flexibility of Exchanges

The term *exchange* refers to a specified, measured amount of food. One exchange does not necessarily indicate a serving; an exchange is simply a precise measure of a food that, when traded for another measured food within the same food group, will yield a similar amount of calories, carbohydrate, protein, and fat. Substituting any food within a food group for another food in the list will give you an even trade. You can think of this concept like receiving a shirt as a gift in a particular style and then exchanging it for one of the same price and size in another style that better suits your preference. Both shirts are the same price and are used for the same purpose, but you prefer one to the other.

You need to become familiar with the foods and their respective measurements for one exchange. When you know the amount in one exchange, you can choose accordingly. For example, bread is in the grains and starches food group. One slice of bread will yield a similar amount of carbohydrate, protein, fat, and calories as any one of the following: one-half of an English muffin, one 6-inch (15-centimeter) diameter tortilla, 3/4 cup (21 grams) of unsweetened, ready-to-eat cereal, 1/2 cup (121 grams) of cooked grits, or 1/2 cup (82 g) of corn. In other words, you may trade one slice of bread for any one of the other items on the list in the amount specified for one exchange.

If you need to make multiple choices from one group, you have several options. If your meal pattern calls for three grains and starches exchanges at a given meal or snack, you have three options:

- Select three different foods in the amount listed for one exchange. For example, you might choose one 6-inch (15-centimeter) corn tortilla, 1/2 cup (82 grams) of corn, and 1 cup (205 grams) of acorn squash.
- Select two different foods, one of which is double the amount for one exchange and one of which is in the amount of one exchange. You could choose 1 cup (164 grams) of corn and 1 cup (205 grams) of acorn squash.
- Select one food in the amount of three exchanges. For example, you could choose 1 1/2 cups (246 grams) of corn.

Foods in Multiple Food Groups

Some foods need to be counted as members of two food groups because of their nutrient content. In other words, they do not fit well into one food group because they supply more nutrients than the typical foods on the list. For example, dried beans, such as black beans, as well as dried peas and lentils are listed under the grains and starches group because they contain a similar amount of carbohydrate as other foods on that list. Additionally, they have more protein than other foods found on that list. Because of their high protein content, they count as one grains and starches exchange and one lean protein exchange (see table 13.2).

One example of a multigroup food that provides the nutrients of more than one food group is sausage. One ounce (30 grams) of chorizo sausage contains approximately 7 grams of protein and 11 grams of fat. Compared with a food on the lean protein list such as skinless turkey breast, which contains 7 grams of protein and 0 to 3 grams of fat, one exchange of chorizo provides an extra 8 to 11 grams of fat. Therefore, chorizo is counted as one lean protein exchange and two fats and oils exchanges because its protein

TABLE 13.2

Multigroup Foods

Food*	FOOD GROUPS		
	Grains and starches	Lean protein	Fats and oils
American cheese, 1 oz (30 g)		1	2
Chorizo, 1 oz (30 g)		1	2
Cornbread, 2 in. (5 cm) cube	1		1
Dried black beans, cooked, 1/2 cup (86 g)	1	1	
Multigrain whole-wheat crackers, 1 oz (30 g)	1		1
Peanut butter, 2 1/2 tbsp (40 g)		1	5

*These foods contain nutrient profiles similar, but not identical, to the foods in the food group in which they are categorized.

content is the same as one exchange of lean protein and its fat content is similar to two fats and oils exchanges.

Peanut and other nut butters are examples of foods that can fall into more than one food group depending on the amount consumed. Each 1/2 tablespoon (8 grams) is one fat and oil exchange until consumption exceeds 2 tablespoons (32 grams). If the amount is greater than 2 tablespoons (32 grams) then enough protein is provided to also count as one lean protein exchange. Thus, 1 tablespoon (16 grams) of nut butter is two fats and oils exchanges, however, 2 1/2 tablespoons provides five fats and oils exchanges and one lean protein exchange. A distinction is made because smaller amounts do not contain sufficient protein to count as a lean protein exchange. In practice, when nut butters are used sparingly as a spread, such as a thin spread of peanut butter on a slice of toast, the amount is usually small and the nut butter counts only toward fats and oils exchanges. When nut butters are used as filling in sandwiches, as part of homemade smoothies, in large amounts on toast, or as the main protein source in a vegetarian dish, the quantity is typically larger and the amount of protein is substantial enough to be accounted for. The amount that you consume, and thus the nutrient profile, determines whether or not the nut butter is a multigroup food.

Knowing that foods are placed into food groups according to their nutrient profiles makes it easier to understand why a food is listed in a particular food group. Although avocados are fruits of the avocado tree, they are counted as fats and oils exchanges because they contain primarily fat, not carbohydrate. Cheese is made from milk, so its protein content causes it to be listed as lean protein, but its fat content counts as a fats and oils exchange. Although plantain is a fruit, 1/3 cup (51 grams) is counted as a grains and starches exchange. Potatoes are thought of as a vegetable, but they are listed in the grains and starches list because of their nutrient content. You need to read the foods in each list carefully to learn where they fit.

Mixed Dishes and Combination Foods

Many foods are made from ingredients that are listed in several food groups. Pizza is an example of such a food. The crust is made from flour, which is in the grains and starches group, and the tomato sauce is in the nonstarchy vegetables group. A pizza may also include cheese, sausage, pepperoni, or ham, items that are counted as both lean protein and fats and oils exchanges. Some pizzas contain fruits such as pineapple or apples. Depending on how much fruit is on the pizza, those ingredients may count as a fruits exchange. As you examine a combination food, ask yourself in which food group the ingredients belong and estimate the amount that you consume. The exchange equivalents for some sample combination foods are shown in table 13.3.

TABLE 13.3

Combination Foods and Their Exchange Equivalents

Combination foods	EXCHANGE EQUIVALENTS		
	Carbohydrate	Protein	Fat
1 1/2 cups (about 250 g) Hoppin' John (black-eyed peas, rice, tomatoes, and sausage)	2 grains and starches (rice, beans)	1 lean protein (sausage)	3 fats and oils (fat from sausage and oil)
	1 nonstarchy vegetables (tomatoes)		
1 shredded beef and cheese burrito (tortilla, beef, cheese, and red chili pepper sauce)	4 grains and starches (tortilla)	1 1/2 lean protein (beef and cheese)	2 fats and oils (fat in the beef and cheese)
	1 nonstarchy vegetables (red sauce)		
1 slice 14 in. (36 cm) sausage pizza (crust, tomato sauce, sausage, and cheese)	2 grains and starches (crust)	2 lean protein (sausage and cheese)	2 fats and oils (fat in sausage, cheese)
	1 nonstarchy vegetables (tomato sauce)		

Customizing Your Meal Plan and Meal Pattern

Humans are creatures of habit. We tend to develop routines and follow the same behavior patterns each day. Over time, routine behaviors become habits. If behavior patterns are counterproductive, however, we have to make adjustments. Creating a meal pattern provides a framework for developing eating habits that support your training, conditioning, and performance goals. The precision meal planning system is

■ flexible, so that you can eat a variety of foods;

- personal, so that you can eat the foods that you like;
- precise, because the correct proportions of carbohydrate, protein, and fat are embedded in the system; and
- calorie controlled, so that you can meet your goal of gaining muscle, losing body fat, or both.

This section guides you through the process of converting the meal plan that you chose in chapter 10, 11, or 12 into a pattern for all your meals and snacks. Your meal plan will look similar to the sample in table 13.4, although the number of exchanges will vary depending on the quantity of calories that you need and your body-composition goals. You decide the number of times that you will eat daily and then distribute your daily allotment of exchanges across those meals and snacks. Your meal plan becomes the framework on which you will select foods and plan your menus, so post it in a highly visible place. Remember that the meal plan is the total number of exchanges for a day. The meal pattern is how you distribute those exchanges across the day as meals and snacks.

TABLE 13.4

Sample 3,600-Calorie Meal Plan

GOALS: GAIN MUSCLE MASS AND LOSE BODY FAT SIMULTANEOUSLY		
Macronutrient	**Food groups**	**Total daily exchanges**
Carbohydrate	Fat-free milk and yogurt	2
	Nonstarchy vegetables	7
	Fruits	13
	Grains and starches	16
	Foods with sugar	3
Protein	Lean protein	8
Fat	Fats and oils	15

Keep the following points in mind as you allocate the exchanges to meals and snacks:

- Eat five or six times a day.
- Eat breakfast.
- Have a snack after exercise that contains carbohydrate and protein.
- Depending on your training, you may also need a preexercise carbohydrate snack.
- Eat most of your food before dinner.

- Eat all the allotted exchanges daily, not more and not less, to increase the likelihood that you will meet your goals.
- Choose fruits, vegetables, and whole grains for fiber to help you feel full.

You should distribute your exchanges throughout the day. Avoid clumping all your foods into a narrow time frame, say from late afternoon to late night. Some research has found an association between eating breakfast and healthy body weight. This finding makes sense when you consider that the body is more active in the early part of the day and will use more calories for energy at that time.

After a meal, some calories are used immediately. Calories that are not immediately used are converted to and stored as fat. Remember, the preferred fuel for moderate- and high-intensity exercise is carbohydrate, not fat! Therefore, during your most intense work periods, you are using mostly carbohydrate, not your stored fat. One way to help keep body weight under control is to eat most of your calories during your most active periods of the day when you store fewer calories as body fat.

The sample meal pattern shown in figure 13.1 is designed for gaining muscle and losing body fat. A pre- and postexercise snack is planned to

FIGURE 13.1   Sample Meal Pattern

3,600-kcal meal plan to build muscle and lose fat

Macronutrients	Food groups	Total daily exchanges	Breakfast	Snack
Carbohydrate	Fat-free milk and yogurt	2	1	
	Nonstarchy vegetables	7		
	Fruits	13	3	2
	Grains and starches	16	4	
	Foods with sugar	3		
Protein	Lean protein	8	1	
Fat	Fats and oils	15	5	

support these training goals. Most of the exchanges are planned before dinner so that you consume the majority of your calories during the most active part of your day, when you burn more of your calories and store fewer calories as fat.

Now you should create your own precision meal pattern using the worksheet shown in figure 13.2. You will need the jumpstart meal plan that you chose in chapter 10, 11, or 12 and the food lists on pages 220 to 233 to guide you. First transfer the total number of exchanges from your meal plan to the column labeled "total daily exchanges." The next step is to distribute your exchanges sensibly among your meals and snacks. Use a pencil because distributing the exchanges across the day requires some trial and error.

Design your meal pattern according to your training routine and your weight and body-composition goals. Make sure to plan the bulk of your food intake in the earlier and most active parts of your day to ensure that you have adequate fuel available during active periods and in optimal proximity to your workouts. Timing of food intake has an effect on how your body uses and stores energy, replenishes nutrients, and recovers from exercise.

Lunch	Preexercise snack	Postexercise snack	Dinner	Snack
		1		
3			4	
3	2	1	2	
3	2	2	5	
	2			1
3			4	
4		2	4	

FIGURE 13.2 Daily Meal Pattern Worksheet

_____ kcal meal plan to _____ *(build muscle, lose fat, or build muscle and lose fat)*

Macronutrients	Food groups	Total daily exchanges	Breakfast	Snack	
Carbohydrate	Fat-free milk and yogurt				
	Nonstarchy vegetables				
	Fruits				
	Grains and starches				
	Foods with sugar				
Protein	Lean protein				
Fat	Fats and oils				

From M. Macedonio and M. Dunford, 2009, *The Athlete's Guide to Making Weight* (Champaign, IL: Human Kinetics). For electronic versions of this form, please visit www.humankinetics.com/TheAthletesGuidetoMakingWeight.

Planning Menus With Your Precision Meal Pattern

After you have created your meal pattern, you use that pattern to plan menus. To simplify this process, work with one meal or snack at a time. In planning your menus consider food preparation time, proximity to your workouts, digestibility, and a reasonable distribution of foods from each of the food lists throughout the day. Begin the day with a well-balanced breakfast to ignite your metabolism after a night's fast. Distribute your protein foods among breakfast, lunch, and dinner, with small amounts at snacks. You can think of snacks as small meals that you should generally consume before and after workouts. In addition to some protein, be sure that your snacks contain carbohydrate from fruits and grains and starches and are low in fat and oils. Liquids digest more quickly than solids do, so you may wish to include smoothies, yogurts, milk, or juices before and after your workouts. This may also be a good time to ingest foods with sugar, such as sports drinks.

The sample menus that follow use the exchange allowances for each meal and snack in the 3,600-calorie meal pattern example in figure 13.1. Remember that each food group list includes many different foods; these menus are only examples. By reviewing the sample meals and snacks, you will get an idea about how to translate the number of exchanges in your meal pattern to actual meals and snacks.

Lunch	Preexercise snack	Postexercise Snack	Dinner	Snack (optional)

Sample Breakfast Menu

English muffins spread with peanut butter, orange juice, and strawberries with fat-free yogurt

Exchange notes:

- ■ 4 oz (120 ml) juice + 4 (120 ml) oz juice + 15 strawberries = 3 fruits exchanges
- ■ 2 English muffins = 4 grains and starches exchanges because 1/2 English muffin is 1 grains and starches exchange

Food and amount	Number of exchanges and food group
8 oz (240 g) fat-free yogurt	1 fat-free milk and yogurt
8 oz (240 ml) orange juice and 15 medium-sized strawberries	3 fruits
2 English muffins	4 grains and starches
2 1/2 tbsp (40 g) peanut butter	5 fats and oils + 1 lean protein

Sample Snack Menu

Large banana or orange

Exchange notes:

■ 1 large piece of fruit = 2 fruits exchanges because 1 small piece of fruit is 1 fruits exchange

Food and amount	Number of exchanges and food group
1 large banana or large orange	2 fruits

Sample Lunch Menu

Ham sandwich, reduced-fat mayonnaise, lettuce, and tomato slices; lettuce salad with raw vegetables, avocado, dried cranberries, and reduced-fat dressing; baked tortilla chips and tomato salsa; large apple; calorie-free beverage such as water, diet soda, sugar-free lemonade, or tea

Exchange notes:

■ 1 large piece of fruit = 2 fruits exchanges because 1 small piece of fruit is 1 fruits exchange

■ 2 slices of bread = 2 grains and starches exchanges because one slice of bread is 1 grains and starches exchange

■ 2 tbsp reduced-fat mayonnaise = 2 fats and oils exchanges because 1 tbsp of reduced-fat mayonnaise is 1 fats and oils exchange

Food and amount	Number of exchanges and food group
1 cup (56 g) lettuce, 1 cup (150 g) chopped raw vegetables, and 1/4 cup (65 g) tomato salsa	3 nonstarchy vegetables
1 large apple, 2 tbsp (15 g) dried cranberries	3 fruits
2 slices whole-grain bread, 1 oz (30 g) bag of baked tortilla chips	3 grains and starches
3 oz (90 g) sliced, lean deli ham	3 lean protein
2 tbsp (28 g) reduced-fat mayonnaise, 1/2 (2 tbsp or 29 g) small avocado, and 2 tbsp (32 g) reduced-fat salad dressing	4 fats and oils

Sample Preexercise Snack Menu

Grapes, graham crackers, sports drink

Exchange notes:

■ 34 grapes = 2 fruits exchanges because 17 grapes is 1 fruits exchange

- 6 graham cracker squares = 2 grains and starches exchanges because 3 squares is 1 grains and starches exchange
- 16 oz (480 ml) sports drink = 2 foods with sugar exchanges because 8 oz (240 ml) is 1 foods with sugar exchange

Food and amount	Number of exchanges and food group
34 grapes	2 fruits
6 graham cracker squares	2 grains and starches
16 oz (480 ml) sports drink	2 foods with sugar

Sample Postexercise Snack Menu

Quick and easy Cheerios cereal mix (see recipe) and low-fat kefir (drinkable yogurt)

This snack contains the carbohydrate and protein that supports muscle growth.

Exchange notes:

- 1 1/2 cup (42 g) Cheerios = 2 grains and starches exchanges because 3/4 cup (21 g) is 1 grains and starches exchange
- 12 almonds = 2 fats and oils exchanges because 6 almonds is 1 fats and oils exchange

Food and amount	Number of exchanges and food group
8 oz (240 ml) low-fat kefir	1 fat-free milk and yogurt
2 tbsp (18 g) raisins	1 fruits
1 1/2 cups (42 g) Cheerios	2 grains and starches
12 almonds	2 fats and oils

Quick and Easy Cheerios Cereal Mix

12 roasted almonds

1 1/2 cups (42 g) Cheerios (any variety)

2 tbsp (18 g) raisins, dried cranberries, or dried blueberries

1. Spread almonds in a single layer on a cookie sheet and roast at 350 degrees Fahrenheit (177 degrees Celsius) for approximately 5 to 10 minutes. Cool completely.
2. Combine almonds with cereal and dried fruit. Store in an airtight container.

Sample Dinner Menu

Grilled marinated, boneless, skinless chicken breast; baked beans; corn; salad with vegetables and dressing; unsweetened applesauce; dinner roll with margarine; calorie-free beverage

Exchange notes:

- 2 cups (112 g) dark green lettuce = 2 nonstarchy vegetables exchanges because 1 cup (56 g) is 1 nonstarchy vegetables exchange
- 2 cups (~300 g) of chopped raw vegetables = 2 nonstarchy vegetables exchanges because 1 cup (~150 g) is 1 nonstarchy vegetables exchange
- 1 cup (244 g) unsweetened applesauce = 2 fruits exchanges because 1/2 cup (122 g) is 1 fruit exchange
- 1 cup (249 g) baked beans = 3 grains and starches exchanges because 1/3 cup (83 g) is 1 grains and starches exchange due to the amount of sugar that is added
- 4 tbsp (64 g) reduced-fat salad dressing = 2 fats and oils exchanges because 2 tbsp (32 g) is 1 fats and oils exchange
- 2 tsp (10 g) margarine = 2 fats and oils exchanges because 1 tsp (5 g) is 1 fats and oils exchange

Food and amount	Number of exchanges and food group
2 cups (112 g) dark green lettuce and 2 cups (~300 g) chopped raw vegetables such as broccoli, tomatoes, carrots, peppers, and radishes	4 nonstarchy vegetables
1 cup (244 g) unsweetened applesauce	2 fruits
1 cup (249 g) baked beans, 1/2 cup (82 g) corn, and 1 whole-grain dinner roll	5 grains and starches
4 oz (120 g) grilled marinated chicken breast	4 lean protein
4 tbsp (64 g) reduced-fat salad dressing and 2 tsp (10 g) margarine	4 fats and oils

Sample Evening Snack Menu

Frozen 100-percent fruit juice bar

Food and amount	Number of exchanges and food group
1 (3 oz or 90 g) frozen 100% fruit juice bar	1 foods with sugar

As you can see, the precision meal planning system provides a great deal of variety and flexibility. When you have committed your meal pattern to memory, you can be confident that by following it you will consume the right amount of energy (calories), and the optimum balance of macronutrients, at the best times to support your training program. Using the food lists gives you the flexibility that you need to choose from the foods available at the time. For instance, when you are at a restaurant, you can easily choose from items on the menu and stay within your meal pattern. The following example illustrates how the same meal pattern can result in two very different dinners.

Same Pattern, Different Menu

Sample dinner menu #1: marinated chicken breast; lettuce salad with vegetables and dressing; unsweetened applesauce; baked beans; dinner roll with margarine

Sample dinner menu #2: shrimp stir fry with vegetables, pineapple, and peanuts over rice

SAMPLE DINNER MENU #1 Food and amount	Number of exchanges and food group	SAMPLE DINNER MENU #2 Food and amount
2 cups (112 g) dark green lettuce and 2 cups (~300 g) broccoli, tomatoes, carrots, peppers, and radishes	4 nonstarchy vegetables	1/2 cup (75 g) cooked red peppers, 1/2 cup (75 g) cooked green peppers, 1/4 cup (16 g) pea pods, 1/4 cup (31 g) water chestnuts, and 1/2 cup (35 g) mushrooms
1 cup (244 g) unsweetened applesauce	2 fruits	1 cup (249 g) canned pineapple
1 cup (249 g) baked beans, 1/2 cup (82 g) corn, 1 whole-grain dinner roll	5 grains and starches	2 1/2 cups (465 g) steamed white rice
4 oz (120 g) grilled marinated chicken breast	4 lean protein	4 oz (120 g) shrimp
4 tbsp (64 g) reduced-fat salad dressing, 2 tsp (10 g) margarine	4 fats and oils	1 tbsp (15 g) peanut oil (for cooking) and 10 peanuts

Menu Ideas for Precision Meals

This section presents a variety of menu ideas for precision meals to help you get started. Design your meals using your meal pattern, but be creative in choosing your foods. For instance, try a breakfast sandwich to add some variety to your meals. Whip up a fruit and yogurt shake or add vegetables to your egg to make an omelet. Remember that you can plan multiple exchanges in several ways. The combinations of foods are endless. The more familiar you are with the precision food lists, the more creative you will be in planning your meals. Remember that the number of exchanges in your meal pattern dictates portion sizes.

Breakfast Menu Ideas

Breakfast is an often-overlooked meal, but beginning the day with ample energy is important, particularly when you have morning practices. Time is a premium in an athlete's schedule, so a bit of planning and preparation will help ensure that you are off to a strong start in the morning with minimal time and effort. If possible include exchanges from fat-free milk and yogurt, fruits, grains and starches, and a modest amount of lean protein and fats and oils. These menu ideas are based on the 3,600-kilocalorie pattern, but you can adjust portions to any calorie level.

- Orange juice; oatmeal with skim milk, raisins, and cinnamon; hard-cooked egg whites and whole-wheat toast with margarine
- English muffin sandwich with Canadian bacon or lean ham; ready-to-eat cereal with skim milk and sliced banana; fruit juice
- Whole-grain bagel, egg, and cheese breakfast sandwich; fat-free yogurt; fruit and nut trail mix; 100-percent fruit juice blend
- Low-fat granola cereal with strawberries or banana and skim milk; scrambled egg and toast with margarine; fruit juice
- Pancakes or waffles with blueberries; poached egg; pineapple juice; skim milk
- French toast (made with egg and milk) topped with mixed berries; fat-free yogurt; orange juice
- Yogurt and fruit shake (see recipe) topped with low-fat granola; whole-grain toast with peanut butter
- English muffin pizza made with shredded part-skim mozzarella cheese, tomato sauce, and pineapple chunks; fruit and nut trail mix; skim milk
- Soy milk smoothie with mango and blueberries; large bagel with sunflower butter and cream cheese
- Feta cheese; melon slices and grapes; pita bread with hummus; olives

Yogurt and Fruit Shake

1 banana (the riper the better)

1 cup (240 g) fat-free yogurt or 1 cup (240 ml) low-fat kefir

1/2 cup (120 ml) orange juice

1 cup (256 g) fresh or frozen fruit (berries, peaches, kiwi, pineapple, mango, cantaloupe)

- -

Combine ingredients and blend until smooth.

Lunch and Dinner Menu Ideas

When planning menus for lunch and dinner, consider whether you will eat meals at home or away, the food options at hand, the need for refrigeration or warming, and preparation time. A well-stocked pantry broadens your menu options, especially when preparing last-minute meals. Healthful varieties of canned, boxed, and frozen foods along with some fresh products allow you a great deal of flexibility when preparing meals. Some menu items can be prepared in quantities large enough to be eaten on several occasions, saving you time and effort. If you routinely eat lunch or dinner in restaurants, take time to preview the menus of your favorite restaurants and preselect several meal options that fit your meal pattern. Being prepared is the key to choosing well.

The menu selections that follow are based on the 3,600-kilocalorie pattern (portions can be adjusted to any calorie level) and offer ideas for meals prepared from scratch and meals created by incorporating prepared foods.

- Hummus with raw vegetables; string cheese and whole-grain crackers; fresh fruit; skim milk (cow's or soy)
- Hummus and vegetable wrap on whole-wheat tortilla (spinach leaves, cucumber, zucchini, onions); apple slices with vanilla yogurt ricotta dip and low-fat granola
- Pizza bagel (whole-grain bagel halves with tomato sauce, onions, lean ham, and part-skim mozzarella); mixed greens salad with low-fat Italian dressing; orange wedges; skim milk
- Tuna, apple, and walnut salad (see recipe) on mixed greens; whole-grain roll; fresh fruit; skim milk (cow's or soy)

Tuna, Apple, and Walnut Salad

6 oz (180 g) tuna packed in water
1 small apple, finely chopped
1 stalk celery, finely chopped
1/2 small onion, finely chopped
2 tbsp (16 g) roasted walnuts, coarsely chopped
2 tbsp (30 g) light mayonnaise
2 tbsp (30 g) fat-free plain yogurt
2 tbsp (30 g) pickle relish
2 tsp (10 g) Dijon mustard
Ground black pepper, onion powder, and garlic powder (optional)

- -

1. Combine all ingredients and mix well.
2. Season to taste with pepper, onion powder, and garlic powder.

Yogurt Ranch Dressing

Reduced-fat ranch dressing   Garlic powder

Plain, nonfat yogurt   Onion powder

1. Combine equal parts ranch dressing and yogurt.
2. Add garlic and onion powder to taste.

- Whole-grain bagel with crunchy peanut butter and sliced bananas; raw vegetables with yogurt ranch dressing (see recipe); skim milk (cow's or soy)
- Turkey sandwich on rye bread with low-fat coleslaw; carrots, grape tomatoes, and sliced peppers with yogurt ranch dressing; cantaloupe with fat-free vanilla yogurt
- Chicken or beef fajita burrito (grilled chicken or beef strips, grilled onions, peppers, and tomatoes and shredded reduced-fat cheese on whole-grain tortilla); baked tortilla chips with chunky tomato–mango salsa; canned peaches with vanilla fat-free yogurt
- Lean roast beef and Swiss cheese on whole-wheat bread with lettuce, tomato, cucumber, and horseradish sauce; fresh pear; skim milk
- Chunky vegetable soup with pasta and grated Romano cheese; almond butter and whole-grain crackers; banana; fat-free yogurt
- Salmon salad and whole-grain crackers; grape tomatoes, carrots, celery, and sliced peppers with yogurt ranch dip; fresh orange; skim milk
- Chicken quesadilla (whole-wheat tortilla, refried beans, grilled onions and peppers, sliced tomatoes, grilled chicken strips, shredded reduced-fat cheese, shredded lettuce); fresh fruit salad; fat-free yogurt
- Chili con carne made with lean beef, tomatoes, beans, and spices served over rice; cabbage slaw with oil and vinegar dressing; cornbread; apple; skim milk
- White chicken chili made with green chilies served over rice; baked tortilla chips and salsa; raw carrots; fresh fruit slices with yogurt dip; skim milk
- Light and lean tuna noodle casserole (see recipe) made with whole-wheat noodles; steamed broccoli and cauliflower; fresh fruit salad; skim milk
- Turkey burger on whole-grain bun with lettuce, tomato, and onion; low-fat coleslaw; grapes; skim milk
- Savory lean hamburgers (see recipe on page 218) on whole-grain bun; seasoned oven-fried sweet potato wedges; mixed green salad with reduced-fat dressing; fresh fruit; skim milk

Light and Lean Tuna Noodle Casserole

12 oz (360 g) extra-wide whole-grain, yolk-free noodles

2 7-oz (210 g) cans or vacuum bags of albacore or chunk light tuna packed in water, drained

1 can 98% fat-free cream of mushroom or cream of celery soup

1/3 cup (75 g) reduced-fat or fat-free mayonnaise

1/2 cup (128 g) evaporated skim milk or 1 cup (240 ml) skim milk

1 cup (182 g) frozen mixed vegetables, cooked

4 oz (120 g) 2% milk Velveeta cheese

4 oz (120 g) jar of chopped pimientos, drained

2 ribs of celery, diced

1 small onion, diced, or 1 tbsp dried onion, or 1 tsp onion powder

Lemon zest or 1 packet of True Lemon lemon powder

1 cup (28 g) whole-grain flake cereal (Corn Flakes, Special K, Total)

1/2 cup (46 g) sliced almonds

Vegetable spray (e.g., Pam)

Liquid margarine spray

1. Preheat oven to 350 degrees Fahrenheit (177 degrees Celsius). Boil egg noodles according to package directions; drain.

2. In a pot, stir together all ingredients except the almonds, cereal, and noodles over low heat until well combined and the cheese has melted.

3. Fold in egg noodles until sauce is evenly distributed. Pour into casserole dish lightly sprayed with vegetable cooking spray. Bake for 30 minutes and sprinkle top with flake cereal and sliced almonds.

4. Add a light spray of liquid margarine over cereal. Bake 10 more minutes until cereal and almonds are lightly browned.

- Pasta and tomato sauce with freshly grated Romano or Parmesan cheese; lean meatballs; romaine and mixed green salad with tomato and low-fat Italian dressing; fresh fruit

- Chicken Parmigiana with linguine (breaded chicken cutlets baked with tomato sauce and topped with shredded mozzarella served with linguine and tomato sauce); mixed green salad; fresh fruit; skim milk

- Chicken stir-fry with vegetables served over brown rice; cucumber salad; fresh fruit with vanilla yogurt

- Barbequed chicken fried rice made with brown rice, carrots, scallions, peas, and green beans; mixed green salad with reduced-fat dressing; baked apple with raisins and cinnamon topped with vanilla yogurt

Savory Lean Hamburgers

1 lb (450 g) 96% lean ground beef (96/4 beef)
1/4 cup (61 g) liquid egg substitute or 2 egg whites (to reduce cholesterol), or
   1 whole egg
1 small onion, chopped
2 tsp (11 g) Worcestershire sauce
2 tsp (10 g) ketchup
1/4 tsp (.7 g) garlic powder

1. Mix all ingredients except garlic powder until well blended, and form into four patties. Sprinkle each patty with garlic powder and lightly pat garlic powder into the meat.
2. Cook on a grill or grill pan on the stovetop to desired doneness.

■ Grilled citrus salmon; brown rice pilaf with slivered almonds; grilled balsamic vinaigrette–marinated zucchini and yellow squash; grilled pineapple slices; skim milk

■ Baked tilapia topped with balsamic vinaigrette–marinated tomatoes and onions; sautéed spinach with garlic and olive oil; baked sweet potato with cinnamon sugar; mixed greens and vegetable salad; canned pears; skim milk

■ Chicken and rice bake (see recipe); tossed green salad; fresh berries; skim milk

■ Asparagus frittata, or omelet, made with part-skim mozzarella cheese; grape tomatoes; whole-grain toast or English muffin with margarine; cantaloupe and fresh strawberries with fat-free vanilla yogurt (The frittata works well with the asparagus stems. You can serve the asparagus tips as a side dish. If you do not care for asparagus, substitute your favorite vegetable.)

■ Rotisserie turkey breast; mashed potatoes with margarine and milk; green beans with garlic and olive oil; mixed greens and romaine lettuce salad with reduced-fat dressing; poached pear; skim milk

■ Orange-glazed lean ham steak; mashed sweet potatoes with cinnamon and margarine (made with fresh or canned sweet potatoes); sweet and sour red cabbage; tossed salad with reduced-fat dressing; cinnamon applesauce; skim milk

■ Oven-fried chicken (coat with flaked cereal crumbs and baked); spicy roasted potato wedges; southern-style greens (collards, turnip greens, or kale); low-fat coleslaw; watermelon; skim milk

Chicken and Rice Bake

4 cups (780 g) cooked brown rice

2 cups (428 g) cooked skinless, white-meat chicken pieces

1 8-oz (240 g) can water chestnuts

1 cup (182 g) mixed (frozen) vegetables, cooked

1 cup (128 g) raw carrots, chopped or shredded

2 cups (240 g) chopped celery

2 medium onions, chopped

3 hard-cooked low-cholesterol eggs, chopped

1/2 cup (112 g) reduced-fat mayonnaise

1/2 cup (120 g) nonfat, plain yogurt

1/2 cup (120 ml) skim milk

1 10-oz can (300 g) reduced-fat cream of chicken soup

Frosted flakes for topping

Vegetable spray (e.g., Pam)

1. Preheat oven to 350 degrees Fahrenheit (177 degrees Celsius).

2. In a large bowl, combine the first eight ingredients (rice, chicken, vegetables, and eggs).

3. In a separate bowl, mix the mayonnaise, yogurt, milk, and soup. Add this mixture into the large bowl and blend well.

4. Pour the entire mixture into a 9 in. by 13 in. (23 by 33 cm) casserole dish that has been sprayed with vegetable spray. Bake for 30 to 45 minutes.

4. During the last 10 minutes, remove the pan from the oven and sprinkle frosted flakes on top of the rice and chicken mixture. Continue cooking for 10 minutes or until slightly browned on top.

Fat-Free Milk and Yogurt Food Group

One fat-free milk and yogurt exchange provides approximately 12 grams of carbohydrate, 8 grams of protein, and 0 to 3 grams of fat.

Each fat-free milk and yogurt exchange includes the following nutrients:

- Simple carbohydrate
- Protein
- Fat, if not skimmed or fat-free
- Vitamins A and D
- B vitamins, particularly riboflavin (B_2)
- Calcium

Precision points:

- Choose fat-free (skim) or low-fat (1%) dairy products to minimize saturated fat and cholesterol. These have 0 to 3 grams of fat per exchange.
- Reduced-fat (2%) varieties count as one fat-free milk and yogurt exchange and one fats and oils exchange because of the extra fat.
- Full-fat (whole) dairy products count as one fat-free milk and yogurt exchange and two fats and oils exchanges because of the amount of fat.
- Evaporated milk has half the water of fresh milk but all the nutrients. It can be used in recipes to bolster milk intake.

Fat-Free Milk and Yogurt

Food	Measurement for 1 exchange
Fat-free (skim) or 1% (low-fat) fluid milk	1 cup (8 oz or 240 ml)
Soy milk, low-fat with added vitamins A and D, and calcium (note: protein, calcium, and vitamin D contents are not as high as cow's milk)	1 cup (8 oz or 240 ml)
Fat-free evaporated milk	1/2 cup (4 oz or 120 ml)
Fat-free powdered milk	1/3 cup (0.8 oz or 23 g) dry powder
Low-fat kefir	1 cup (8 oz or 240 ml)
Yogurt, fat-free, plain or artificially sweetened	6 oz (180 g)
Yogurt, low-fat, plain or artificially sweetened	6 oz (180 g)

Reduced-Fat and Whole Milk

Food	Measurement for exchanges
FOODS COUNTING AS 1 FAT-FREE MILK AND YOGURT EXCHANGE AND 1 FATS AND OILS EXCHANGE	
2% (reduced-fat) fluid milk	1 cup (8 oz or 240 ml)
Soy milk, enriched with calcium and vitamins A and D	1 cup (8 oz or 240 ml)
2% (reduced-fat) evaporated milk	1/2 cup (4 oz or 120 ml)
FOODS COUNTING AS 1 FAT-FREE MILK AND YOGURT EXCHANGE AND 2 FATS AND OILS EXCHANGES	
Whole fluid milk	1 cup (8 oz or 240 ml)
Whole evaporated milk	1/2 cup (4 oz or 120 ml)

Nonstarchy Vegetables Food Group

One nonstarchy vegetables exchange provides approximately 5 grams of carbohydrate, 2 grams of protein, and 0 grams of fat.

Each nonstarchy vegetables exchange includes the following nutrients:

- Complex carbohydrate
- Protein
- A variety of vitamins and minerals; some are high in the antioxidants, vitamins A and C
- Fiber (except for vegetable juice)

Precision points:

- One cup (~150 g) raw is about the size of a Wiffleball baseball.
- 1/2 cup (~75 g) cooked is amount in an ice cream scoop or a baseball cut in half.
- Without added sauces or fats, vegetables are low in calories and high in nutrients, so precise measurement is not necessary.
- Some canned vegetables and vegetable juices are high in sodium because of processing.

Nonstarchy Vegetables

Food	
Artichoke	Mixed vegetables without corn, peas, or pasta
Artichoke hearts	Mushrooms
Asparagus*	Okra
Beans (green, wax, Italian)	Onions
Bean sprouts	Parsley
Beets	Parsnips
Broccoli**	Peppers*
Brussels sprouts**	Radishes
Cabbage*	Salad greens (romaine*, leaf lettuce, Boston lettuce)
Carrots	Sauerkraut
Cauliflower**	Summer squash* (yellow crookneck squash)
Celery	Tomato*
Cucumber	Tomatoes, canned
Eggplant	Tomato sauce, fat-free or very low fat
Green onions or scallions	Tomato or vegetable juice**
Greens* (collard, endive, escarole, kale**, mustard, spinach, Swiss chard, turnip)	Turnips
	Water chestnuts
Kohlrabi* (stem turnip)	Watercress
Leeks	Zucchini
Lettuce (dark green leafy*)	

*Good source of vitamin C: 6 mg-11-mg per serving

**Excellent source of vitamin C: 12 mg or more per serving

Fruits Food Group

One fruit exchange provides approximately 15 grams of carbohydrate and 0 grams of protein and fat.

Each fruits exchange includes the following nutrients:

- Simple and complex carbohydrate
- A variety of vitamins and minerals, some high in vitamin C; some juices are fortified with vitamins and minerals
- Fiber (except for fruit juice)

Precision points:

- A piece of fruit that is one fruits exchange is about the size of a tennis ball.
- 1/2 cup (~125 g) serving is the size of a baseball cut in half.
- Choose unsweetened when possible.
- When appropriate, eat with skin. Wash well before eating.

Fruits

Food	Measurement for 1 exchange
Apple, unpeeled	1 small (4 oz or 120 g)
Applesauce, unsweetened	1/2 cup (122 g)
Apples, dried	4 rings
Apricots, fresh	4 whole
Apricots, dried	8 halves
Apricots, canned, no sugar added	1/2 cup (126 g)
Banana	1 small (4 oz or 120 g)
Berries: blackberries, blueberries, boysenberries, raspberries*, sliced strawberries**	1 cup (144 g)
Strawberries **, whole	1 1/4 cup (180 g) or 15 medium berries
Cantaloupe**	1 cup (177 g) cubes or balls or 1/3 small melon
Cherries, sweet, fresh	15
Cherries, sweet, canned, water-packed	1/2 cup (124 g)
Clementine (tangerine)**	2 small
Cranberries, dried	2 tbsp (15 g)
Dates, deglet noor	3
Dates, medjool	1
Figs, fresh	1 large or 2 medium (3.5 oz or 105 g)
Figs, dried	3
Fruit cocktail, canned, water-packed	1 cup (237 g)

Fruits Food Group

Food	Measurement for 1 exchange
Fruit cocktail, canned, light syrup	1/2 cup (121 g)
Grapefruit*	1/2 large (11 oz or 330 g)
Grapes	17 small
Guava**	1/2 cup (82 g)
Honeydew melon	1 cup cubes or balls or 1/10 of a medium melon (5 oz or 134 g)
Kiwi**	1 large (3 oz or 90 g)
Mandarin oranges*, juice-packed	2/3 cup (167 g)
Mango**	1/2 cup (3 oz or 90 g)
Nectarine	1 small, 2 1/2 in. (6 cm) diameter
Orange**	1 small, 3 in. (7.5 cm) diameter
Papaya**	1/2 medium (5 in. or 13 cm) or 1 cup (140 g) cubes
Peach, fresh	1 medium (3 in. or 7.5 cm) diameter
Peaches, canned, juice-packed	1/2 cup (125 g)
Pear, fresh	1/2 large (3.5 oz or 100 g)
Pears, canned, juice-packed	1/2 cup (124 g)
Pineapple, fresh**	3/4 cup (116 g)
Pineapple*, canned, juice-packed	1/2 cup (124 g)
Plums, fresh	2 small (6 oz or 180 g)
Plums, canned, juice-packed	1/2 cup (125 g)
Plums, dried (prunes)	3
Raisins	2 tbsp (18 g)
Tangerines (mandarin orange), fresh**	1 large (2 3/4 in. or 7 cm diameter)
Watermelon**	1 1/4 cup cubed or balls, 1 wedge, or 7 oz (210 g)
FRUIT JUICE	
Apple juice or cider	1/2 cup (120 ml)
Cranberry juice cocktail**	See foods with sugar
Fruit juice blends, 100% juice**	1/3 cup (80 ml)
Grape juice	1/3 cup (80 ml)
Grapefruit juice**	1/2 cup (120 ml)
Orange juice**	1/2 cup (120 ml)
Pineapple juice*	1/2 cup (120 ml)
Prune juice	1/3 cup (80 ml)

*Good source of vitamin C: 6 mg–11 mg per serving
**Excellent source of vitamin C: 12 mg or more per serving

Grains and Starches Food Group

One grains and starches exchange provides approximately 15 grams of carbohydrate, 0 to 3 grams of protein, and 0 to 1 gram of fat

Each grains and starches exchange includes the following nutrients:

■ Complex and simple carbohydrates

■ B-complex vitamins

■ Fiber—in whole grains, beans, and starchy vegetables

■ Protein—in beans, peas, lentils, small amount in grains

■ The antioxidants vitamin E and selenium—in whole grains

Precision points:

■ General rule: 1 ounce (30 grams) of a grain product is one exchange.

■ One cup is the size of a baseball or the fist of an average adult.

■ 1/2 cup is the size of a baseball cut in half or the amount in an ice cream scoop.

■ A medium potato is the size of a small computer mouse.

■ A 3-ounce (90-gram) bagel is approximately 3 inches (7.5 centimeters) in diameter, or the size of a hockey puck.

■ Choose 100% whole grain when possible.

■ Choose low-fat grains and starches when possible.

Grains and Starches

Food	Measurement for 1 exchange
BREADS	
Bagel	1/2 small (2 oz or 60 g; 3 in. or 7.6 cm) or 1/3 medium (3 oz or 90 g; 4 in. or 10.2 cm) or 1/4 bakery sized (4 oz or 120 g; 5 in. or 12.7 cm)
Bread, reduced-calorie	2 slices
Bread (whole grain, multigrain, whole wheat, rye, pumpernickel, white)	1 slice (1 oz or 30 g)
Bread sticks, crisp, 7 1/2 in. by 1/2 in. (20 cm by 1.3 cm)	2 sticks (2/3 oz or 20 g)
English muffin	1/2
English muffin, reduced-calorie	1
Hot dog bun or hamburger bun	1/2
Pancake, 4 in. (10 cm) across, 1/4 in. (0.6 cm) thick	1
Pita, 6 in. (15 cm) across	1/2
Roll, plain dinner	1 small (1 oz or 30 g)
Raisin bread, unfrosted	1 slice (1 oz or 30 g)
Tortilla, corn or flour, 6 in. (15 cm) across	1
Tortilla, flour, 10 in. (25 cm) across	1/3
Tortilla, flour, 13 in. (33 cm) across	1/4

Grains and Starches Food Group

Food	Measurement for 1 exchange
Waffle, 4 in. (10 cm) across, reduced-fat	1
CEREALS AND GRAINS	
Bran cereal	1/2 cup (20 g)
Bulgur wheat, cooked	1/2 cup (91 g)
Cereals, cooked with water (oatmeal, grits, cream of wheat)	1/2 cup (121 g)
Cereals, unsweetened, ready-to-eat	3/4 cup (21 g)
Cereals, sweetened, ready-to-eat	1/2 cup (20 g)
Granola, low-fat	1/4 cup (27 g)
Grape Nuts	1/4 cup (29 g)
Kasha	1/2 cup (84 g)
Muesli	1/4 cup (21 g)
Oats, dry	1/3 cup (51 g)
Pasta, rice, couscous—cooked	1/2 cup (~ 70 g of pasta or 93 g of rice)
Puffed cereal	1 1/2 cup (33 g)
Wheat germ	3 tbsp (22 g)
STARCHY VEGETABLES	
Baked beans	1/3 cup (83 g)
Corn	1/2 cup (82 g) or 1/2 large cob (5 oz or 150 g)
Mixed vegetables with corn, peas, carrots	1 cup (150 g)
Peas, green	1/2 cup (72 g)
Plantain	1/3 cup (51 g)
Potato, boiled	1/2 cup (3 oz or 90 g) or 1/2 medium
Potato, baked or roasted with skin	1/2 cup (3 oz or 90 g) or 1/4 large potato
Squash, winter, baked (acorn, butternut, pumpkin)	1 cup (205 g)
Yam, sweet potato, plain	1/2 cup (100 g) 1 medium (4 oz or 114 g) 1/2 large (7 oz or 198 g)
CRACKERS AND SNACKS	
Graham cracker, 2 1/2 in. (6 cm) square	3
Oyster crackers	20
Popcorn (popped, no fat added, or low-fat microwave)	3 cups (24 g)
Pretzels	3/4 oz (21 g)
Saltine-type crackers	7
Whole-wheat crackers, no fat added, saltine type	7 (3/4 oz or 21 g)
Triscuit, whole-grain crackers, reduced-fat	5 (3/4 oz or 20 g)

Grains and Starches Food Group

Beans, Peas, and Lentils

Food	Measurement for exchanges
FOODS COUNTING AS 1 GRAINS AND STARCHES EXCHANGE AND 1 LEAN PROTEIN EXCHANGE	
Beans and peas (black, black-eyed, garbanzo, Great Northern, kidney, lima, navy, pinto), cooked	1/2 cup (100 g)
Lentils	1/2 cup (96 g)
Miso (soybean paste)	3 tbsp (52 g)

Grains and Starches Prepared With Fat

Food	Measurement for exchanges
FOODS COUNTING AS 1 GRAINS AND STARCHES EXCHANGE AND 1 FATS AND OILS EXCHANGE	
Biscuit	1 small (2 1/2 in. or 6 cm)
Chow mein noodles	1/2 cup (22 g)
Croutons	1/2 cup (20 g)
Crackers, round butter type	6
French fries, oven-baked (see fast foods list for fried)	1 cup (50 g) or 10 fries
Granola, regular	1/4 cup (30 g)
Hummus (garbanzo puree)	1/3 cup (81 g)
Muffin (such as banana, blueberry, bran)	1 oz (30 g) or 1/5 bakery sized
Popcorn with butter or oil, microwaved	3 cups (24 g)
Ramen noodles	1/2 package (1 oz or 28 g)
Sandwich crackers (peanut butter or cheese filling)	3
Snack chips (potato, tortilla)	9–13 chips (3/4 oz or 21 g)
Stuffing, bread (prepared)	1/3 cup (66 g)
Taco shell, 6 in. (15 cm) across	2
Waffle, 4 in. (10 cm) square or across	1
Whole-wheat crackers	2–5 (3/4 oz or 20 g)

Foods With Sugar Food Group

One exchange of foods with sugar provides approximately 15 grams of carbohydrate. Depending on the food choice an exchange may include some protein and fat. The food list notes which foods contain exchanges for other food groups (for example, fats and oils or fat-free milk and yogurt).

Foods with sugar generally lack vitamins, minerals, and fiber but are sources of carbohydrate, primarily simple (refined) carbohydrate. Items in the foods with sugar group may contain one or more of the following nutrients:

- Protein, depending on the ingredients
- Fat, depending on the ingredients; may be significant and may have concentrated amounts of saturated and trans fats
- Vitamins and minerals, if these nutrients have been added

Precision points:

- Some foods are more nutritious than others. For instance, pudding made with fat-free milk has a higher nutrient density than cookies with creme filling.
- Athletes often choose foods with sugar as part of pre- or postexercise snacks.

Foods With Sugar Counting as One Exchange

Food	Measurement for 1 exchange
Barbeque sauce	3 Tbsp (1.8 oz or 51 g)
Chocolate chip cookie, small *Also count as 2 fats and oils exchanges*	2 (2 1/4 inch across)
Cranberry juice cocktail	1/2 cup (120 ml)
100% fruit juice bar, frozen	1 bar (3 oz or 90 g)
Fruit snacks, chewy (pureed fruit)	1 roll (3/4 oz or 21 g)
Fruit spread, 100% fruit	1 1/2 tbsp (27 g)
Gelatin, regular, prepared with water	1/2 cup (135 g)
Gingersnaps	3
Honey	1 tbsp (21 g)
Hot chocolate, regular, made with 8 oz (240 ml) water *Also counts as 1 fats and oils exchange*	1 envelope (1 oz or 28 g)
Hot chocolate, sugar-free or light, made with 8 oz (240 ml) water	1 envelope (0.6 oz or 16 g)
Ice cream, light *Also count as 1 fats and oils exchange*	1/2 cup (71 g)
Jam or jelly	1 tbsp (21 g)
Milk, chocolate, fat-free or low-fat *Also counts as 1 fat-free milk and yogurt exchange*	1 cup (8 oz or 240 ml)
Rice drink, plain, fat-free	1 cup (8 oz or 240 ml)

(continued)

Foods With Sugar Food Group

Foods With Sugar Counting as One Exchange, *continued*

Food	Measurement for 1 exchange
Rice drink, flavored, low-fat	1/2 cup (4 oz or 120 ml)
Salad dressing, fat-free or low-fat, cream-based	3 tbsp (48 g)
Sports drink	1 cup (8 oz or 240 ml)
Sugar	1 tbsp (12 g)
Syrup, light	2 tbsp (42 g)
Syrup, regular	1 tbsp (21 g)
Trail mix, candy- or nut-based *Also counts as 2 fats and oils exchanges*	1 oz (30 g)
Trail mix, dried fruit-based *Also counts as 1 fats and oils exchange*	1 oz (30 g)
Yogurt, frozen, fat-free	1/3 cup (48 g)
Yogurt, frozen, regular, soft serve *Some brands count as 1 fats and oils exchange*	1/2 cup (72 g)

Foods With Sugar Counting as One-and-a-Half Exchanges

Food	Measurement for 1 1/2 exchanges
Cranberry sauce, jellied	1/4 cup (69 g)
Doughnut, plain cake *Also counts as 2 fats and oils exchanges*	1 medium (1 1/2 oz or 45 g)
Energy gel	1 oz (30 g) or 1 packet
Energy, sport, meal replacement, or breakfast bar *Some brands count as 1 fats and oils exchange*	1 1/3 oz (40 g) bar
Granola or snack bar, regular or low-fat	1 oz (30 g) bar
Ice cream, fat-free, no sugar added	1/2 cup (71 g)
Pie, pumpkin or custard *Also counts as1 1/2 fats and oils exchanges*	1/8 of 8-in. (20 cm) pie
Pudding, fat-free, prepared	1/2 cup (4 oz or 113 g)

Foods With Sugar Food Group

Foods With Sugar Counting as Two Exchanges

Food	Measurement for 2 exchanges
Angel food cake, unfrosted	1/12 of cake (~2 oz or 60 g)
Cake, frosted *Also counts as 1 fats and oils exchange*	2-in. (5 cm) square (~2 oz or 60 g)
Chocolate chip cookie, bakery type *Also count as 2 fats and oils exchanges*	1 3 in. (1.6 oz or 45 g)
Cupcake, frosted *Also counts as 1–1 1/2 fats and oils exchanges*	1 small (~2 oz or 60 g)
Doughnut, yeast type, glazed *Also counts as 2 fats and oils exchanges*	3 3/4 in. (9.5 cm) across (2 oz or 60 g)
Energy, sport, meal replacement or breakfast bar *Also counts as 1 fats and oils exchange*	2 oz (60 g) bar
Energy drink	1 can (8.3 oz or 250 ml)
Fruit drink or lemonade	1 cup (8 oz or 240 ml)
Pudding, regular, prepared with reduced-fat milk	1/2 cup (140 g)
Sherbet, sorbet	1/2 cup (74 g)
Ice cream, fat-free	1/2 cup (71 g)

Foods With Sugar Counting as Two-and-a-Half Exchanges

Food	Measurement for 2 1/2 exchanges
Brownie, unfrosted, *Also count as 1 fats and oils exchange*	2-in. (5 cm) square (2 oz or 60 g)
Brownie, frosted *Also count as 2 fats and oil exchanges*	1 1/2-in. (3.8 cm) square (1.5 oz or 51 g)
Soft drink (soda), regular	1 can (12 oz or 360 ml)
Sweet roll or Danish *Also counts as 2 fats and oils exchanges*	2 1/2 oz (75 g)

Foods With Sugar Counting as Three Exchanges

Food	Measurement for 3 exchanges
Fruit cobbler *Also counts as 1 fats and oils exchange*	1/2 cup (3 1/2 oz or 105 g)
Pie, fruit, 2 crusts *Also counts as 2 fats and oils exchanges*	1/6 of 8-in. (20 cm) pie

Lean Protein Food Group

One lean protein exchange provides approximately 7 grams of protein and 0 to 3 grams of fat.

Each lean protein exchange includes the following nutrients:

- Protein
- Some B vitamins, especially riboflavin (B_2), niacin (B_3), and B_{12}
- Iron (except dairy products)

Precision points:

- One ounce (30 grams) of lean protein is the size of a 9-volt battery, a matchbook, two dominoes, or four dice.
- Three ounces (90 grams) of meat, fish, or poultry is about the size of a deck of cards, a bar of soap, or a checkbook.
- Eight ounces (240 grams) of meat, fish, or poultry is about the size of a thin paperback book.
- One tablespoon (16 grams) of nut butter is the size of half of a walnut shell. Two tablespoons (32 grams) is the size of a Ping-Pong ball.
- Check the label for fat content and choose the leanest (lowest fat) products. Aim for 3 grams of fat per ounce (per 30 grams) or less.
- Anything greater than 3 grams of fat per ounce (per 30 grams) should be counted as one fat exchange for each additional 5 grams of fat. For example, 1 ounce (30 grams) of protein food that contains 8 grams of fat equals one lean protein exchange and one fats and oils exchange.
- Traditionally processed meats (sausage, hot dogs, and deli meats such as bologna, pepperoni, salami) and cheese are extremely high in fat, saturated fat, cholesterol, and sodium.
- Cooking method affects fat content and calories. Low-fat methods include baking, boiling, stewing, broiling, grilling, poaching, and steaming. Avoid breaded and fried versions.
- Peanut and other nut butters are high-fat proteins. The fat is heart-healthy.
- Animal products are sources of cholesterol and saturated fats. Limit total cholesterol to 300 milligrams per day or less.

Lean Protein Food Group

Lean Protein

Food	Measurement for 1 exchange
Beef, lean cuts, trimmed: round, sirloin, flank steak, tenderloin, or filet	1 oz (30 g)
Beef jerky	1 oz (30 g)
Canadian bacon or lean ham	1 oz (30 g)
Cheese (parmesan or Romano), grated	2 tbsp (10 g)
Cheese, low-fat (3 g fat or less per oz, or per 30 g)	1 oz (30 g)
Chicken or turkey, skinless, white or dark meat	1 oz (30 g)
Cold cuts and sandwich meats, 98% fat-free (3 g fat or less per oz, or per 30 g)	1 oz (30 g)
Cottage cheese	1/4 cup (56 g)
Egg whites	2
Egg substitute, plain, liquid	1/4 cup (61 g)
Fish or shellfish, fresh or canned (clams, crab, lobster, scallops, shrimp)	1 oz (30 g)
Game (buffalo, ostrich, rabbit, venison), skinless	1 oz (30 g)
Hot dog, reduced-fat (1 g fat per oz or per 30 g)	1 oz (30 g)
Other meats (pork, veal, lamb): roasts, chops, trimmed loin or tenderloin	1 oz (30 g)
Oysters, fresh or frozen	6 medium
Salmon, canned	1 oz (30 g)
Sausage, reduced-fat (1 g fat per oz or per 30 g)	1 oz (30 g)
Tuna, canned in water or oil, drained	1 oz (30 g)

Protein Foods With Fat

Food	Measurement for exchanges
FOODS COUNTING AS 1 LEAN PROTEIN EXCHANGE AND 1 FATS AND OILS EXCHANGE	
Egg, yolk and white	1 large
Cheese, regular	1 slice (1 oz or 30 g)
Mozzarella, part-skim	1 oz (30 g)
Ricotta cheese, part-skim	1/4 cup (2 oz or 60 g)
Sausage with 5 g fat	1 oz (30 g)
Tempeh (soybean cake)	1/4 cup (42 g)
Tofu	1/2 cup or 4 oz (120 g)
FOODS COUNTING AS 1 LEAN PROTEIN EXCHANGE AND 5 FATS AND OILS EXCHANGES	
Peanut butter or almond butter	2 1/2 tbsp (40 g)

Fats and Oils Food Group

One fats and oils exchange provides approximately 5 grams of fat.

Nutrients:

■ Fat. The type of fat may be saturated or unsaturated.

■ Plant fat supplies vitamin E.

■ Nuts and seeds supply some protein and fiber.

Precision points:

■ One tablespoon (16 grams) of nut butter is the size of half of a walnut shell. Two tablespoons (32 grams) is the size of a Ping-Pong ball.

■ Fat is high in calories. Measure quantities carefully and do not exceed the number of exchanges in your plan.

■ Whenever possible, choose heart-healthy monounsaturated or polyunsaturated fat, which is found in plant fat.

■ Animal products are sources of cholesterol and saturated fat. Limit total cholesterol to 300 milligrams or less per day.

■ Peanut butter and other nut butters are high in fat. When used in small quantities (up to 2 tablespoons, or 32 grams) as a spread they are counted as fats and oils exchanges. In larger quantities, the protein is accounted for by adding one lean protein exchange.

Fats and Oils Food Group

Fats and Oils

Food		Measurement for 1 exchange
HEART-HEALTHY FATS		
Avocado		1/2 small or 2 tbsp (29 g)
Margarine	Regular	1 tsp (5 g)
	Reduced-fat	1 tbsp (15 g)
Mayonnaise	Regular	1 tsp (5 g)
	Reduced-fat	1 tbsp (14 g)
Miracle Whip	Regular	2 tsp (11 g)
	Reduced-fat	1 tbsp (16 g)
Oil		1 tsp (5 g)
Olives	Ripe (black)	8 large
	Green, stuffed	10 large
Nuts, almond, cashews		6 nuts
Mixed nuts or peanuts		10 nuts
Pecan halves		4 halves
Peanut butter, almond butter, cashew butter		1/2 tbsp (8 g)
Salad dressing	Regular	1 tbsp (16 g)
	Reduced-fat	2 tbsp (32 g)
Seeds (flaxseed, sesame, sunflower, pumpkin)		1 tbsp (8 g)
Tahini (sesame seed paste)		2 tsp (10 g)
SATURATED FATS (CONTAIN CHOLESTEROL)—LIMIT CONSUMPTION		
Bacon, pork or turkey		1 slice (1/2 oz or 15 g)
Butter		1 tsp (5 g) or 1 pat
Whipped butter		2 tsp (6 g)
Cream, half and half		2 tbsp (30 g)
Cream cheese	Regular	1 tbsp (1/2 oz or 14 g)
	Reduced-fat (Neufchatel)	1 1/2 tbsp (3/4 oz or 23 g)
Sour cream	Regular	2 tbsp (29 g)
	Reduced-fat or light	3 tbsp (45 g)

Appendix A

Additional Resources

ACTIVITY CALCULATORS

www.shapeup.org—On the Shape Up America! Web site, click on Resource Center and look for the Physical Activity Calculator.

www.nutristrategy.com—This Web site provides a chart that lists the calories burned during different types of exercise. It also has nutrition and fitness software available for purchase.

www.mypyramid.gov—On this Web site from the United States Department of Agriculture, you can use the MyPyramid Tracker. Click on MyPyramid Tracker and look for the Assess Your Physical Activity link.

NUTRIENT ANALYSIS PROGRAMS

The following open access programs are free, but their databases may be limited or the sites may be slow because of heavy traffic.

www.mypyramid.gov—The United States Department of Agriculture offers the MyPyramid Tracker. Click on MyPyramid Tracker and look for the Assess Your Food Intake link.

www.shapeup.org—At Shape Up America!, click on Resource Center and look for the Meal and Snack Calculator.

www.nat.uiuc.edu—NAT version 2.0 is provided by the Food Science and Human Nutrition Department at the University of Illinois.

The following programs are available for purchase. These comprehensive programs allow users to add specialty foods and recipes to the database, but both the initial program and updates cost money and require a thorough understanding of foods and preparation methods.

www.esha.com—ESHA provides a program called Food Processor.

www.nutritionco.com—The Nutrition Company offers a program called Food-works.

www.axxya.com—Nutritionist Pro is created by Axxya Systems.

www.nutribase.com—NutriBase sells a program called NutriBase 7.

RESISTANCE TRAINING

www.acsm.org—The American College of Sports Medicine Web site. Click on Resources for the General Public and then click on Brochures. Scroll down to the brochures available as pdf files. The brochure topics include selecting and effectively using free weights and home weights.

Aaberg, E. 2006. *Muscle mechanics.* 2nd ed. Champaign, IL: Human Kinetics.

Stoppani, J. 2006. *Encyclopedia of muscle and strength.* Champaign, IL: Human Kinetics.

RESTING METABOLIC RATE CALCULATOR

www.shapeup.org—Click on Resource Center of the Shape Up America! site and look for the Resting Metabolic Rate Calculator.

SUPPLEMENTS

www.cfsan.fda.gov—The Center for Food Safety and Applied Nutrition, which helps to carry out the mission of the Food and Drug Administration, provides recent information on supplements. Under the program area, click on the Dietary Supplements link.

VITAMINS AND MINERALS

http://fnic.nal.usda.gov—For more information about vitamins and minerals, visit the Food and Nutrition Information Center of the USDA's National Agriculture Library. Click on Dietary Guidance and follow the Dietary Reference Intakes (DRI) links.

http://www.iom.edu/Object.File/Master/21/372/0.pdf—This link takes you to charts from the Institute of Medicine that provide more information about daily intake and the tolerable upper intake levels of vitamins and minerals.

Appendix B

Tools and Templates

The following tips, forms, and lists will help you determine and record your daily food intake and activity. These items will help you to track and assess your diet and and your exercise energy expenditure accurately as well as to monitor changes in weight and body composition.

To assist you in planning meals and snacks that will help you to meet your weight and body composition goals, exchanges are included for popular menu items available at fast food restaurants and for products that have been specially formulated for athletes. Use this information as part of the precision meal planning system explained in chapter 13.

Track Your Progress

Weight and body-composition goal: _____

Date	Age	Height		RMR	Total Weight		Weight Change			Body Fat				Lean Mass		
		in.	cm		lb	kg	lb	kg	%	%	lb	kg	Change +/-	lb	kg	Change +/-

From M. Macedonio and M. Dunford, 2009, *The Athlete's Guide to Making Weight* (Champaign, IL: Human Kinetics). For electronic versions of this form, please visit www.humankinetics.com/TheAthletesGuidetoMakingWeight

Food Intake Record

Date _____

Name _____ Weight _____ Height _____

Time or meal	Food item and method of preparation	Amount eaten

From M. Macedonio and M. Dunford, 2009, *The Athlete's Guide to Making Weight* (Champaign, IL: Human Kinetics). For electronic versions of this form, please visit www.humankinetics.com/TheAthletesGuidetoMakingWeight.

Additional Tips for Recording Food Intake

Record everything that you eat and drink for the next three to seven days in the amounts that you consumed. Record the foods and beverages that you consume as soon as possible afterward while the information is fresh in your memory. The accuracy of your assessment depends on the accuracy of your records. The following guidelines can help you produce accurate records.

Be Specific

- ☐ Use brand names when you know them. Refer to the Nutrition Facts label on the package, if possible.
- ☐ Indicate whether the food is fresh, canned, or frozen.
- ☐ If the food is canned or frozen, note whether it was packed in water, oil, or syrup.
- ☐ If the product is frozen, indicate whether it was breaded.
- ☐ Record whether the food had gravy or sauce.
- ☐ Note the preparation method: baked, fried, grilled, broiled, sautéed, steamed, boiled, and so forth.
- ☐ List any additions made in preparation: butter, oil, margarine, milk, cream, eggs, nuts, seeds, and so on.
- ☐ If you eat food from a restaurant (fast-food or sit-down style), list the restaurant name.

Estimate Portion Sizes Correctly

- ☐ Use standard measures: cups, tablespoons, teaspoons, ounces (milliliters, grams).
- ☐ Use these portions guidelines to help with your estimates:
  - ▪ 3 ounces (90 grams) meat = the size a deck of cards
  - ▪ Medium apple or orange = the size of a tennis ball
  - ▪ 1/2 cup nonliquid food = the size of a tennis ball
  - ▪ 1/2 cup (4 oz or 120 ml) liquid = the amount in a cone-shaped paper cup
  - ▪ 1 cup non-liquid food = the size of a baseball
  - ▪ 1 cup (8 oz or 240 ml) liquid = 1/2-pint carton of milk
  - ▪ Gatorade bottle = 20 ounces (600 ml)

Don't Forget the Extras

- ☐ Condiments: Note what you added and how much.
  - ▪ Mayonnaise: light or regular?
  - ▪ Ketchup, mustard, steak sauce, or salsa.
  - ▪ Salad dressing: regular or reduced-fat? Note the brand.
  - ▪ Sour cream, butter, or margarine: regular or reduced-fat?
  - ▪ Cream or sugar.
- ☐ Record other miscellaneous items.
  - ▪ Bread or rolls: white, whole wheat, rye, or raisin?
  - ▪ Bagels or tortillas: whole grain or white? Indicate ounces (grams) or diameter.
  - ▪ Milk: white or chocolate? Whole, 2%, 1%, skim (fat free), or soy?
  - ▪ Coffee or tea: regular or decaf?
  - ▪ Soda pop: regular or sugar free?
  - ▪ Desserts: Be as specific as possible.

From M. Macedonio and M. Dunford, 2009, *The Athlete's Guide to Making Weight* (Champaign, IL: Human Kinetics). For electronic versions of this form, please visit www.humankinetics.com/TheAthletesGuidetoMakingWeight.

Activity Record

Record your activities and the actual time spent exercising each day for the next seven days. You may want to do this when you record your seven-day food intake. You can also enter each activity into an online calculator or the nutrient analysis program you used to calculate the calories consumed from food.

Time	Minutes spent exercising	Minutes spent in other activities (sleep, deskwork, etc.)	Intensity
12:00 a.m.			
1:00 a.m.			
2:00 a.m.			
3:00 a.m.			
4:00 a.m.			
5:00 a.m.			
6:00 a.m.			
7:00 a.m.			
8:00 a.m.			
9:00 a.m.			
10:00 a.m.			
11:00 a.m.			
12:00 p.m.			
1:00 p.m.			
2:00 p.m.			
3:00 p.m.			
4:00 p.m.			
5:00 p.m.			
6:00 p.m.			
7:00 p.m.			
8:00 p.m.			
9:00 p.m.			
10:00 p.m.			
11:00 p.m.			

From M. Macedonio and M. Dunford, 2009, *The Athlete's Guide to Making Weight* (Champaign, IL: Human Kinetics). For electronic versions of this form, please visit www.humankinetics.com/TheAthletesGuidetoMakingWeight.

Fast Food and the Precision Meal Planning System

The choices in the fast-food list are approximations of common selections at fast-food or chain restaurants. The exchanges below were calculated based on the *ingredients* and the *nutrient composition* of the menu items as supplied by the restaurant Web sites. Due to differences in ingredients used by restaurants and in home cooking, the exchanges listed do not exactly match those in the Precision Food Lists. Specific nutrition information for most restaurants is available at the restaurant or its Web site.

Fast-Food List

Food	Serving	EXCHANGES		
		Carbohydrate	Protein	Fat
BREAKFAST SANDWICHES				
Egg, cheese, meat, English muffin	1 sandwich	2 grains and starches	2 lean protein	1 fats and oils
Bacon, egg, cheese biscuit	1 sandwich	2 grains and starches	1 lean protein	4 fats and oils
Sausage, egg, biscuit	1 sandwich	2 grains and starches	1 lean protein	6 fats and oils
Hotcakes (3), sausage patty, syrup	1 order	4 grains and starches 3 foods with Sugar	1 lean protein	4 fats and oils
Burrito with sausage	1 sandwich	3 grains and starches	3 lean protein	5 fats and oils
Burrito with steak	1 sandwich	3 grains and starches	3 lean protein	4 fats and oils
ENTRÉES				
Burrito (beef, beans, cheese, onions, tomato, sour cream, lettuce, red sauce tortilla)	1 sandwich	3 grains and starches	1 lean protein	3 fats and oils
Burrito (chicken, beans, cheese, onions, tomato, sour cream, lettuce, red sauce tortilla)	1 sandwich	3 grains and starches	1 1/2 lean protein	2 1/2 fats and oils
Large burrito (13-inch tortilla, carnitas, rice, pinto beans, tomato salsa, lettuce, guacamole, sour cream)	1 burrito	7 grains and starches	5 lean protein	8 fats and oils
Large burrito (13-inch tortilla, chicken, rice, pinto beans, fajita vegetables, tomato salsa, lettuce, guacamole)	1 burrito	8 grains and starches	5 lean protein	5 fats and oils
Large burrito (13-inch tortilla, steak, rice, tomato salsa, corn salsa, sour cream, guacamole)	1 burrito	7 1/2 grains and starches	5 lean protein	7 fats and oils
Chicken breast sandwich—breaded, fried (mayo, tomato, lettuce, bun)	1 sandwich	3 grains and starches	3 lean protein	3 fats and oils
Chicken breast sandwich—grilled (lettuce, tomato, mayo dressing, bun)	1 sandwich	1 nonstarchy vegetables, 3 grains and starches	3 lean protein	1 fats and oils
Chicken breast, breaded, fried	1 breast	1/2 grains and starches	3 lean protein	2 fats and oils
Chicken drumstick, breaded, fried	1 drumstick	1/2 grains and starches	1/2 lean protein	1 fats and oils
Chicken nuggets, breaded, fried	10 pieces	2 grains and starches	3 lean protein	3 fats and oils
Chicken patty sandwich—breaded, fried (bun)	1 sandwich	3 grains and starches	1 lean protein	3 fats and oils
Chicken tenders, breaded	3 pieces	3 grains and starches	4 lean protein	5 fats and oils

(continued)

Fast-Food List, *continued*

Food	Serving	EXCHANGES		
		Carbohydrate	Protein	Fat
Fish patty, breaded, (American cheese, tartar sauce, bun)	1 sandwich	3 grains and starches	1 lean protein	3 fats and oils
Hamburger, single	1 sandwich	2 1/2 grains and starches	2 1/2 lean protein	2 fats and oils
Hamburger, single, with cheese	1 sandwich	2 1/2 grains and starches	3 lean protein	3 fats and oils
Hamburger, double, with cheese	1 sandwich	2 1/2 grains and starches	5 1/2 lean protein	5 fats and oils
ASIAN FOODS				
Fried rice, 8 oz (240 g)	1 dinner	4 1/2 grains and starches		3 fats and oils
Orange chicken	1 dinner	3 grains and starches	2 lean protein	4 fats and oils
Kung pao chicken	1 dinner	1 grains and starches	2 lean protein	2 fats and oils
Mongolian beef	1 dinner	1 grains and starches	1 lean protein	2 fats and oils
Crispy shrimp	1 dinner	2 grains and starches	1 lean protein	2 fats and oils
Sweet and sour pork	1 dinner	1 grains and starches	4 lean protein	2 fats and oils
PIZZA				
Cheese, pepperoni, regular, 14 in. (36 cm)	1/8 of pie	2 grains and starches	1 lean protein	2 fats and oils
Cheese, vegetables, thin crust, 14 in. (36 cm)	1/4 of pie	1 1/2 grains and starches	1 lean protein	2 fats and oils
Cheese, hand-tossed, 14 in. (36 cm)	1/8 of pie	1 1/2 grains and starches	1 lean protein	1 fats and oils
SALAD				
Main dish salad, grilled chicken, greens, vegetables, beans, salad dressing	1 salad	2 nonstarchy vegetables, 2 grains and starches	3 lean protein	1 fats and oils
Main dish Asian salad, grilled chicken, greens, vegetables, fruit, reduced-fat salad dressing	1 salad	2 nonstarchy vegetables, 1 fruits, 1 grains and starches	3 lean protein	1 fats and oils
Side salad, 3 oz (90 g), no cheese, no dressing	1 salad	1 nonstarchy vegetables		
SIDES AND APPETIZERS				
French fries, small	2 1/2 oz (75 g)	2 grains and starches		3 fats and oils
French fries, medium	4 oz (120 g)	3 grains and starches		4 fats and oils
French fries, large	6 oz (180 g)	5 grains and starches		6 fats and oils
Nachos with cheese, small	4.5 oz (135 g)	2 1/2 grains and starches		4 fats and oils
Onion rings, small	3 oz (90 g)	2 1/2 grains and starches		3 fats and oils
DESSERTS				
Vanilla shake, 12 oz (360 g)	1 medium	1 1/2 fat-free milk and yogurt, 5 foods with sugar		3 fats and oils
Vanilla, reduced-fat ice cream cone, 3 oz (90 g)	1 cone	1/2 fat-free milk and yogurt, 1 foods with sugar		1 fats and oils
Fruit and yogurt parfait, 5 oz (150 g)	1 parfait	1/2 fat-free milk and yogurt, 1 foods with sugar		

From M. Macedonio and M. Dunford, 2009, *The Athlete's Guide to Making Weight* (Champaign, IL: Human Kinetics). For electronic versions of this form, please visit www.humankinetics.com/TheAthletesGuidetoMakingWeight.

Products Formulated for Athletes

These products are specially formulated for the nutrient needs of athletes and therefore the nutrient profiles of these products do not fall neatly into one food list. The *ingredient* list and *nutrient composition* of each product were used to calculate the exchange equivalents.

| Product | Serving | EXCHANGES | | |
		Carbohydrate	Protein	Fat
HIGH-PROTEIN RECOVERY AND MEAL REPLACEMENT DRINKS				
Boost High Protein	8 oz (240 g) bottle	1 1/2 fat-free milk and yogurt, 1 foods with sugar		1 fats and oils
Boost Drink	8 oz (240 g) bottle	1 1/2 fat-free milk and yogurt, 1 1/2 foods with sugar		1 fats and oils
Boost Smoothie	8 oz (240 g) bottle	1 1/2 fat-free milk and yogurt, 1 1/2 foods with sugar		1/2 fats and oils
Ensure High Protein	8 oz (240 g) bottle	1 1/2 fat-free milk and yogurt, 1 foods with sugar		1 fats and oils
Ensure	8 oz (240 g) bottle	1 1/2 fat-free milk and yogurt, 1 1/2 foods with sugar		1 fats and oils
Gatorade Nutrition Shake	11 oz (310 g) can	2 fat-free milk and yogurt, 1 1/2 foods with sugar		1/2 fats and oils
Gatorade Protein Recovery Shake	11 oz (310 g) can	2 fat-free milk and yogurt, 2 foods with sugar		1 1/2 fats and oils
Myoplex Powder	78 g packet	1/2 fat-free milk and yogurt, 1/2 grains and starches, 1/2 foods with sugar	5 lean protein	
PROTEIN POWDERS*				
Beneprotein Whey Protein Powder	7 g scoop or 1 packet		1 lean protein	
EAS Whey Protein Powder	1 oz (30 g) scoop		3 lean protein	

*Protein powders vary greatly. Carefully read the Nutrition Facts Label, including the ingredients listing. Whey and casein protein will contain complete protein whereas individual amino acid formulas may not contain all essential amino acids and are therefore incomplete protein.

From M. Macedonio and M. Dunford, 2009, *The Athlete's Guide to Making Weight* (Champaign, IL: Human Kinetics). For electronic versions of this form, please visit www.humankinetics.com/TheAthletesGuidetoMakingWeight.

Works Consulted

American College of Sports Medicine, Armstrong LE, Casa DJ, et al. 2007. American College of Sports Medicine position stand. Exertional heat illness during training and competition. *Medicine and Science in Sports and Exercise*, 39(3):556–572.

American College of Sports Medicine, Sawka MN, Burke LM, et al. 2007. American College of Sports Medicine position stand. Exercise and fluid replacement. *Medicine and Science in Sports and Exercise*, 39(2):377–390.

American College of Sports Medicine. 2008. Sodium balance and exercise. *Current Sports Medicine Reports*, 7(4) Suppl 1:S1–S55.

Armstrong LE, Costill DL, and Fink WJ. 1985. Influence of diuretic-induced dehydration on competitive running performance. *Medicine and Science in Sports and Exercise*, 17(4):456–461.

Baker LB, Conroy DE, and Kenney WL. 2007. Dehydration impairs vigilance-related attention in male basketball players. *Medicine and Science in Sports and Exercise*, 39(6):976–983.

Baker LB, Dougherty KA, Chow M, et al. 2007. Progressive dehydration causes a progressive decline in basketball skill performance. *Medicine and Science in Sports and Exercise*, 39(7):1114–1123.

Blumberg S. 2005. Liar liar: Federal Trade Commission rooting out false diet advertisers. *Journal of the American Dietetic Association*, 105(12):1850–1853.

Chan JL, Heist K, DePaoli AM, et al. 2003. The role of falling leptin levels in the neuroendocrine and metabolic adaptation to short-term starvation in healthy men. *Journal of Clinical Investigation*, 111(9):1409–1421.

Corrigan B, and Kazlauskas R. 2003. Medication use in athletes selected for doping control at the Sydney Olympics (2000). *Clinical Journal of Sport Medicine*, 13(1):33–40.

Cribb PJ, Williams AD, and Hayes A. 2007. A creatine-protein-carbohydrate supplement enhances responses to resistance training. *Medicine and Science in Sports and Exercise*, 39(11):1960–1968.

Cribb PJ, Williams AD, Stathis CG, et al. 2007. Effects of whey isolate, creatine, and resistance training on muscle hypertrophy. *Medicine and Science in Sports and Exercise*, 39(2):298–307.

Deutz RC, Benardot D, Martin DE, et al. 2000. Relationship between energy deficits and body composition in elite female gymnasts and runners. *Medicine and Science in Sports and Exercise*, 32(3):659–668.

Dunford M, and Doyle JA. 2008. *Nutrition for Sport and Exercise*. Belmont, CA: Thomson Wadsworth.

Ebert TR, Martin DT, Bullock N, et al. 2007. Influence of hydration status on thermoregulation and cycling hill climbing. *Medicine and Science in Sports and Exercise*, 39(2):323–329.

Edwards AM, Mann ME, Marfell-Jones MJ, et al. 2007. Influence of moderate dehydration on soccer performance: physiological responses to 45 min of outdoor match-play and the immediate subsequent performance of sport-specific and mental concentration tests. *British Journal of Sports Medicine*, 41(6):385–391.

Garrow JS, and Summerbell CD. 1995. Meta-analysis: Effect of exercise, with or without dieting, on the body composition of overweight subjects. *European Journal of Clinical Nutrition*, 49(1):1–10.

George CF, Kab V, and Levy AM. 2003. Increased prevalence of sleep-disordered breathing among professional football players. *New England Journal of Medicine*, 348(4):367–368.

Gibala MJ, and Howarth KR. 2006. In Dunford M (ed.), *Sports Nutrition: A Practice Manual for Professionals*, pp 33–49. Chicago: American Dietetic Association.

Gruenwald J, Brendler T, and Jaenicke C (eds). 2007. *PDR for Herbal Medicines*, 4th ed. Montvale, NJ: Thomson Healthcare.

Haaz S, Fontaine KR, Cutter G, et al. 2006. Citrus aurantium and synephrine alkaloids in the treatment of overweight and obesity: An update. *Obesity Reviews*, 7(1):79–88.

Halson SL, Lancaster GI, Achten J, et al. 2004. Effects of carbohydrate supplementation on performance and carbohydrate oxidation after intensified cycling training. *Journal of Applied Physiology*, 97:1245–1253.

Harp JB, and Hecht L. 2005. Obesity in the National Football League. *Journal of the American Medical Association*, 293(9):1061–1062.

Heer M, Baisch F, Kropp J, et al. 2000. High dietary sodium chloride consumption may not induce body fluid retention in humans. *American Journal of Physiology, Renal, Fluid and Electrolyte Physiology*, 278(4):F585–F595.

Hinton PS, Sanford TC, Davidson MM, et al. 2004. Nutrient intakes and dietary behaviors of male and female collegiate athletes. *International Journal of Sport Nutrition and Exercise Metabolism*, 14(4):389–405.

Hoffman J, Ratamess N, Kang J, et al. 2006. Effect of creatine and beta-alanine supplementation on performance and endocrine responses in strength/power athletes. *International Journal of Sport Nutrition and Exercise Metabolism*, 16(4):430–446.

Institute of Medicine. 2006. *Dietary Reference Intakes: The Essential Guide to Nutrient Requirements*. Otten JJ, Hellwig JP, and Meyers LD (eds). Washington, DC: National Academies Press.

Keski-Rahkonen A, Kaprio J, Rissanen A, et al. 2003. Breakfast skipping and health-compromising behaviors in adolescents and adults. *European Journal of Clinical Nutrition*, 57(7):842–853.

Kraemer WJ, Torine JC, Silvestre R, et al. 2005. Body size and composition of National Football League players. *Journal of Strength and Conditioning Research*, 19(3):485–489.

Kurpad AV, Muthayya S, and Vaz M. 2005. Consequences of inadequate food energy and negative energy balance in humans. *Public Health Nutrition*, 8(7A):1053–1076.

Lamboley CR, Royer D, and Dionne IJ. 2007. Effects of beta-hydroxy-beta-methylbutyrate on aerobic-performance components and body composition in college students. *International Journal of Sport Nutrition and Exercise Metabolism*, 17(1):56–69.

Laurson KR, and Eisenmann JC. 2007. Prevalence of overweight among high school football linemen. *Journal of the American Medical Association*, 297(4):363–364.

Lundy B, O'Connor H, Pelly F, et al. 2006. Anthropometric characteristics and competition dietary intakes of professional rugby league players. *International Journal of Sport Nutrition and Exercise Metabolism*, 16(2):199–213.

Malina RM, Morano PJ, Barron M, et al. 2007. Overweight and obesity among youth participants in American football. *Journal of Pediatrics*, 151(4):378–382.

Maughan RJ. 2003. Impact of mild dehydration on wellness and on exercise performance. *European Journal of Clinical Nutrition*, 57, Suppl 2:S19–S23.

McArdle WD, Katch FI, and Katch VL. 2007. *Exercise Physiology: Energy, Nutrition, and Human Performance*, 6th ed. Baltimore: Lippincott Williams & Wilkins.

Miller SL, Tipton KD, Chinkes DL, et al. 2003. Independent and combined effects of amino acids and glucose after resistance exercise. *Medicine and Science in Sports and Exercise*, 35(3):449–455.

Montgomery DL. 2006. Physiological profile of professional hockey players—a longitudinal comparison. *Applied Physiology, Nutrition, and Metabolism*, 31(3):181–185.

National Strength and Conditioning Association (NSCA). 2005. *Performance Training Journal: Baseball and Softball*, 4(1):10–11.

Nogueira JA, and Da Costa TH. 2004. Nutrient intake and eating habits of triathletes on a Brazilian diet. *International Journal of Sport Nutrition and Exercise Metabolism*, 14(6):684–697.

O'Connor DM, and Crowe MJ. 2007. Effects of six weeks of beta-hydroxy-beta-methylbutyrate (HMB) and HMB/creatine supplementation on strength, power, and anthropometry of highly trained athletes. *Journal of Strength and Conditioning Research*, 21(2):419–423.

Onywera VO, Kiplamai FK, Boit MK, et al. 2004. Food and macronutrient intake of elite Kenyan distance runners. *International Journal of Sport Nutrition and Exercise Metabolism*, 14(6):709–719.

Petersen HL, Peterson CT, Reddy MB, et al. 2006. Body composition, dietary intake, and iron status of female collegiate swimmers and divers. *International Journal of Sport Nutrition and Exercise Metabolism*, 16(3):281–295.

Phillips SM, Hartman JW, and Wilkinson SB. 2005. Dietary protein to support anabolism with resistance exercise in young men. *Journal of the American College of Nutrition*, 24(2):134S–139S.

Phillips SM, Moore DR, and Tang JE. 2007. A critical examination of dietary protein requirements, benefits, and excesses in athletes. *International Journal of Sport Nutrition and Exercise Metabolism*, 17(Suppl):S58–S76.

Physicians Desk Reference (PDR) Staff. 2008. *Physicians Desk Reference*, 62nd ed. Montvale, NJ: Thompson PDR.

Rankin JW, Goldman LP, Puglisi MJ, et al. 2004. Effect of post-exercise supplement consumption on adaptations to resistance training. *Journal of the American College of Nutrition*, (4):322–330.

Sawka MN, and Montain SJ. 2000. Fluid and electrolyte supplementation for exercise heat stress. *American Journal of Clinical Nutrition*, 72(2 Suppl):564S–572S.

Secora CA, Latin RW, Berg KE, et al. 2004. Comparison of physical and performance characteristics of NCAA Division I football players: 1987 and 2000. *Journal of Strength and Conditioning Research*, 18(2):286–291.

Sharpe PA, Granner ML, Conway JM, et al. 2006. Availability of weight-loss supplements: Results of an audit of retail outlets in a southeastern city. *Journal of the American Dietetic Association*, 106(12):2045–2051.

Shekelle PG, Hardy ML, Morton SC, et al. 2003. Efficacy and safety of ephedra and ephedrine for weight loss and athletic performance: A meta-analysis. *Journal of the American Medical Association*, 289(12):1537–1545.

Stiegler P, and Cunliffe A. 2006. The role of diet and exercise for the maintenance of fat-free mass and resting metabolic rate during weight loss. *Sports Medicine*, 36(3):239–262.

Strauss RH, Lanese RR, and Malarkey WB. 1985. Weight loss in amateur wrestlers and its effect on serum testosterone levels. *Journal of the American Medical Association*, 254(23):3337–3338.

Terpstra AH. 2004. Effect of conjugated linoleic acid on body composition and plasma lipids in humans: an overview of the literature. *American Journal of Clinical Nutrition*, 79(3):352–361.

Timlin MT, Pereira MA, Story M, et al. 2008. Breakfast eating and weight change in a 5-year prospective analysis of adolescents: Project EAT (Eating Among Teens). *Pediatrics,* 121(3):e638–e645.

Tipton K, Elliott T, Cree M, et al. 2004. Ingestion of casein and whey proteins results in muscle anabolism after resistance exercise. *Medicine and Science in Sports and Exercise,* 36:2073–2081.

Tipton KD, and Wolfe RR. 2004. Protein and amino acids for athletes. *Journal of Sports Sciences,* 22:65–79.

van der Heijden AA, Hu FB, Rimm EB, et al. 2007. A prospective study of breakfast consumption and weight gain among U.S. men. *Obesity (Silver Spring),* 15(10):2463–2469.

Volek JS, and Rawson ES. 2004. Scientific basis and practical aspects of creatine supplementation for athletes. *Nutrition,* 20(7–8):609–614.

Welle S, Matthews DE, Campbell RG, et al. 1989. Stimulation turnover by carbohydrate feeding in men. *American Journal of Physiology,* 257(3 Prt 1), E413–E417.

Wheeler M, Daly A, Evert A, Franz M, et al. 2008. Choose your foods: Exchange Lists for Diabetes. *Journal of the American Dietetic Association,* 108(5): 883-888.

Whigham LD, Watras AC, and Schoeller DA. 2007. Efficacy of conjugated linoleic acid for reducing fat mass: A meta-analysis in humans. *American Journal of Clinical Nutrition,* 85(5):1203–1211.

Williams, M. 2007. *Nutrition for Health, Fitness, and Sport,* 8th ed. New York: McGraw Hill.

Wilmore JH, Costill DL, and Kenney WL. 2008. *Physiology of Sport and Exercise,* 4th ed. Champaign, IL: Human Kinetics.

Yon BA, Johnson RK, Harvey-Berino J, et al. 2007. Personal digital assistants are comparable to traditional diaries for dietary self-monitoring during a weight loss program. *Journal of Behavioral Medicine,* 30(2):165–175.

Yoshida T, Takanishi T, Nakai S, et al. 2002. The critical level of water deficit causing a decrease in human exercise performance: a practical field study. *European Journal of Applied Physiology,* 87(6):529–534.

Index

Note: The italicized *f* and *t* following page numbers refer to figures and tables, respectively.

Y

About the Authors

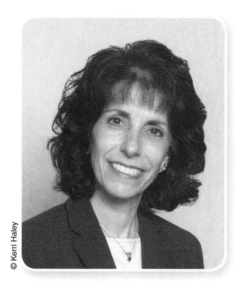

© Kerri Haley

Michele Macedonio, MS, RD, CSSD, LD, a nationally recognized dietitian and board-certified specialist in sport dietetics, is the team dietitian for the Cincinnati Bengals and Cincinnati Reds. A freelance nutrition writer and editor, Macedonio has authored many nutrition articles and educational materials and has contributed chapters to *Sports Nutrition: A Guide for the Professional Working With Active People* (third edition) and *Sports Nutrition: A Practice Manual for Professionals* (fourth edition). She has spent 25 years working on the nutrition of high school, collegiate, and professional athletes and other active people. Macedonio, a frequent lecturer, is the owner of the consulting firm Nutrition Strategies. She is also an active member of Sports, Cardiovascular and Wellness Nutrition (SCAN) and the recipient of their 2007 Achievement Award. She holds master's degrees in health sciences education and nutrition from Case Western Reserve University. Macedonio lives in Loveland, Ohio.

Marie Dunford, PhD, RD, is a freelance nutrition author and editor of nutrition education materials, including textbooks, consumer books, online courses, continuing professional education courses, and magazine and newspaper articles. She is coauthor of the textbook *Nutrition for Sport and Exercise* and editor of *Sports Nutrition: A Practice Manual for Professionals* (fourth edition). A former professor and chair in the department of food science and nutrition at California State University at Fresno, Dunford has extensive experience with NCAA Division I athletes. She is an active member of SCAN and recipient of their 2006 Achievement Award. She received a PhD in education from the University of Southern California

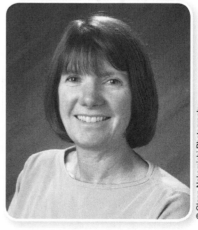

© Glenn Nakamichi Photography

and a master's degree in home economics from California State University at Fresno. Dunford lives in Kingsburg, California, and is an avid tennis player.